MW00846131

Reviews and critical articles covering the entire field of normal anatomy (cytology, histology, cyto- and histochemistry, electron microscopy, macroscopy, experimental morphology and embryology and comparative anatomy) are published in Advances in Anatomy, Embryology and Cell Biology. Papers dealing with anthropology and clinical morphology that aim to encourage cooperation between anatomy and related disciplines will also be accepted. Papers are normally commissioned. Original papers and communications may be submitted and will be considered for publication provided they meet the requirements of a review article and thus fit into the scope of "Advances". English language is preferred.

It is a fundamental condition that submitted manuscripts have not been and will not simultaneously be submitted or published elsewhere. With the acceptance of a manuscript for publication, the publisher acquires full and exclusive copyright for all languages and countries.

Twenty-five copies of each paper are supplied free of charge.

Manuscripts should be addressed to

Prof. Dr. F. **BECK**, Howard Florey Institute, University of Melbourne,
Parkville, 3000 Melbourne, Victoria, Australia
e-mail: fb22@le.ac.uk

Prof. Dr. F. **CLASCÁ**, Department of Anatomy, Histology and Neurobiology,
Universidad Autónoma de Madrid, Ave. Arzobispo Morcillo s/n, 28029 Madrid, Spain
e-mail: francisco.clasca@uam.es

Prof. Dr. M. **FROTSCHER**, Institut für Anatomie und Zellbiologie, Abteilung für Neuroanatomie,
Albert-Ludwigs-Universität Freiburg, Albertstr. 17, 79001 Freiburg, Germany
e-mail: michael.frotscher@anat.uni-freiburg.de

Prof. Dr. D. E. **HAINES**, Ph.D., Department of Anatomy, The University of Mississippi Med. Ctr.,
2500 North State Street, Jackson, MS 39216-4505, USA
e-mail: dhaines@anatomy.umsmed.edu

Prof. Dr. H.-W. **KORF**, Zentrum der Morphologie, Universität Frankfurt,
Theodor-Stern Kai 7, 60595 Frankfurt/Main, Germany
e-mail: korf@em.uni-frankfurt.de

Prof. Dr. E. **MARANI**, Department Biomedical Signal and Systems, University Twente,
P.O. Box 217, 7500 AE Enschede, The Netherlands
e-mail: e.marani@utwente.nl

Prof. Dr. R. **PUTZ**, Anatomische Anstalt der Universität München,
Lehrstuhl Anatomie I, Pettenkoferstr. 11, 80336 München, Germany
e-mail: reinhard.putz@med.uni-muenchen.de

Prof. Dr. Dr. h.c. Y. **SANO**, Department of Anatomy,
Kyoto Prefectural University of Medicine,
Kawaramachi-Hirokoji, 602 Kyoto, Japan

Prof. Dr. Dr. h.c. T.H. **SCHIEBLER**, Anatomisches Institut der Universität,
Koellikerstraße 6, 97070 Würzburg, Germany

# 190
# Advances in Anatomy
# Embryology
# and Cell Biology

Editors

F. F. Beck, Melbourne · F. Clascá, Madrid
M. Frotscher, Freiburg · D. E. Haines, Jackson
H.-W. Korf, Frankfurt · E. Marani, Enschede
R. Putz, München · Y. Sano, Kyoto
T. H. Schiebler, Würzburg

Stefan Britsch

# The Neuregulin-I/ErbB Signaling System in Development and Disease

With 14 Figures and 2 Tables

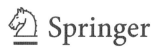 Springer

**Stefan Britsch, Prof. Dr.**

Max Delbrück Centre for Molecular Medicine (MDC) Berlin-Buch
Robert-Roessle-Str. 10
13125 Berlin
Germany

present address:

Georg-August-Universität Göttingen
Zentrum Anatomie
Kreuzbergring 36
37075 Göttingen
Germany

*e-mail: sbritsch@mdc-berlin.de*

Figure on page IX was reproduced with the kind permission of Cold Spring Harbor Laboratory Press.

ISSN 0301-5556
ISBN 978-3-540-37105-2  Springer Berlin Heidelberg New York

This work is subject to copyright. All rights reserved, whether the whole or part of the material is concerned, specifically the rights of translation, reprinting, reuse of illustrations, recitation, broadcasting, reproduction on microfilm or in any other way, and storage in data banks. Duplication of this publication or parts thereof is permitted only under the provisions of the German Copyright Law of September, 9, 1965, in its current version, and permission for use must always be obtained from Springer-Verlag. Violations are liable for prosecution under the German Copyright Law.

Springer is a part of Springer Science+Business Media
springer.com
© Springer-Verlag Berlin Heidelberg 2007

The use of general descriptive names, registered names, trademarks, etc. in this publication does not imply, even in the absence of a specific statement, that such names are exempt from the relevant protective laws and regulations and therefore free for general use.
Product liability: The publisher cannot guarantee the accuracy of any information about dosage and application contained in this book. In every individual case the user must check such information by consulting the relevant literature.

Editor: Simon Rallison, Heidelberg
Desk editor: Anne Clauss, Heidelberg
Production editor: Nadja Kroke, Leipzig
Cover design: WMX Design Heidelberg
Typesetting: LE-TeX Jelonek, Schmidt & Vöckler GbR, Leipzig

# Acknowledgements

The author wishes to thank Carmen Birchmeier for her continuous scientific support. He gratefully acknowledges Alistair Garratt, Hagen Wende, and Marie Trendelenburg, as well as the members of the Birchmeier lab for discussions and critical comments on the manuscript. Work from the author was supported by grants from the DFG.

# List of Contents

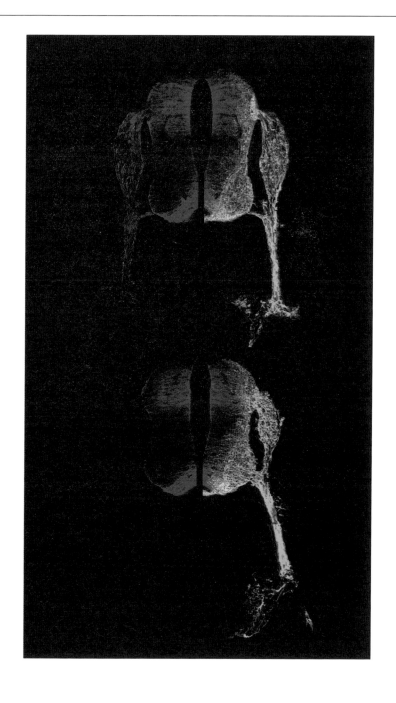

*There is no science without fancy and no art without facts.*
Vladimir Nabokov

# Abbreviations

| | |
|---|---|
| −/− | Homozygous null mutation of a given gene |
| ARIA | Acetylcholine receptor inducing activity |
| BDNF | Brain-derived neurotrophic factor |
| bHLH | Basic helix-loop-helix |
| BMP | Bone morphogenetic protein |
| CNS | Central nervous system |
| CNTF | Ciliary neurotrophic factor |
| CRD | Cysteine-rich domain |
| *Dom* | Dominant megacolon, naturally occurring mutant allele of the Sox10 gene |
| E | Developmental day |
| EGF | Epidermal growth factor |
| ENS | Enteric nervous system |
| ErbB | Derived from avian erythroblastosis tumor virus, the oncogenic variant of the EGFR receptor (= ErbB1) |
| ES | Embryonic stem (cell) |
| FGF | Fibroblast growth factor |
| GDNF | Glial cell line-derived neurotrophic factor |
| GGF | Glial growth factor |
| IGF | Insulin-like growth factor-1 |
| LIF | Leukemia inhibitory factor |
| NCC | Neural crest cell |
| NDF | Neu differentiation factor |
| NRG | Neuregulin |
| NT | Neurotrophin |
| PDGF | Platelet-derived growth factor |
| PNS | Peripheral nervous system |
| RTK | Receptor tyrosine kinase |
| Shh | Sonic hedgehog |
| SMDF | Sensory and motoneuron derived factor |
| Sox | Sry box |
| TGF$\beta$ | Transforming growth factor $\beta$ |
| VEGF | Vascular endothelial cell growth factor |

# 1
# Introduction: Molecular Control of Development

The development of a multicellular organism from the fertilized egg is the result of spatiotemporally orchestrated processes like cell proliferation, migration, differentiation, survival, and death. During evolution general strategies have evolved that allow coordination and tight control of such events over time and space:

- Cell-intrinsic mechanisms, such as cell-autonomous control of gene expression

- Cell-extrinsic mechanisms, such as cell-to-cell communication through secreted signal molecules and their corresponding receptors

Such cell-extrinsic signaling systems may involve the exchange of information between neighboring cells (short range signals), between distant cells or tissues (long range signals), or between cells and the extracellular surrounding space. Conserved signaling pathways, like the Wnt, Shh, TGF-$\beta$, or Delta/Notch pathways form the molecular basis of cell-to-cell communication systems. Characteristically, a limited number of signaling systems is used repeatedly by an individual organism to regulate independent cellular events during embryonic development (Artavanis-Tsakonas et al. 1999; Massague et al. 2000; Peifer and Polakis 2000; Ingham and McMahon 2001; Anderson and Ingham 2003). Shh signals, for example, control via their specific receptors' *patched* and *smoothened* developmental events as diverse as pattern formation in the ventral spinal cord or the formation of teeth (Ingham and McMahon 2001). Particular signaling molecules, like the fibroblast growth factors (FGFs), neurotrophins, and vascular endothelial cell growth factors (VEGF) transmit their signals to target cells via transmembrane receptors of the tyrosine kinase family (Schlessinger 2000). This class of signaling molecules is pioneered by the epidermal growth factor (EGF) and its specific tyrosine kinase receptor EGFR (HER1, or ErbB1).

Tyrosine kinase receptor-mediated signals have been extensively demonstrated to control fundamental biological processes, such as proliferation, survival, migration, and differentiation during development as well as in the adult (Schlessinger 2000). The EGF/ErbB signaling system is evolutionarily highly conserved. Both the nematode *Caenorhabditis elegans*, and the fruit fly *Drosophila melanogaster* have primordial versions of the EGF/ErbB signaling pathway. In higher organisms, this has developed into a complex signaling network. The principle functional features, however, of this signaling system were already defined in invertebrates: EGF/ErbB-mediated signals regulate the fate of diverse cell lineages during different developmental stages through short-range paracrine cell-to-cell interactions. *C. elegans* and *Drosophila* each contain a single ErbB homologue. However, a single EGF-like ligand in C. elegans, *Lin-3*, has evolved into four ligand variants in *Drosophila*, named *Vein*, *Gurken*, *Spitz*, and *Argos*. In *C. elegans* the *Lin-3* ligand is secreted from a gonadal anchor cell. Vulval precursor cells respond to *Lin-3* signals through a transmembrane receptor, *let-23*, and *Lin-3* instructs them to undergo further proliferation and differentiation. The *Lin-3* pathway functions in other morphogenetic processes as well. Loss-of-function mutations not only result in a vulvaless phenotype, but also in sterility, and abnormal male tail development (Aroian et al. 1990; Aroian and Sternberg 1991). The *Drosophila* EGFa receptor *DER* is used repeatedly in different developmental scenarios, like oogenesis, and wing and eye development (Yarden and Sliwkowski 2001). However, different EGF-like ligands are employed, depending on the developmental event. Differentiation of *DER*-expressing tendon cells is regulated by a myotube-derived Neuregulin-like ligand, *Vein* (Yarnitzky et al. 1997; Volk 1999), whereas the TGF-$\alpha$ homologue *Gurken* functions in oocyte development. Neuregulins and TGF-$\alpha$ are both EGF-like ligands in higher vertebrates, where at least 10 different EGF-like ligands and four different EGFR-like molecules have been identified.

Invertebrates like *Drosophila* or *C. elegans* have become indispensable models for studying general functions of conserved signaling systems like the EGF/ErbB signaling pathway. Indeed, much of the progress in understanding vertebrate development has come from the conservation of a relatively small set of signaling pathways defined in flies and worms (Anderson and Ingham 2003). However, studies in invertebrates do not allow the direct analysis of functions that have evolved in parallel to the diversification of ligands as well as their receptor molecules in higher organisms (Yarden and Sliwkowski 2001).

Our understanding of the molecular mechanisms underlying embryonic development in higher organisms has been revolutionized by the availability of genetic techniques that allow the selective disruption and/or modification of a gene (*gene targeting*) in the genome of mouse embryonic stem (ES) cells (Muller 1999; Britsch et al. 2003; Britsch 2006). This has allowed the study of individual genes by specifically altering their functions in vivo. At present, more than 10% of the genes in the mouse genome have been disrupted using *gene targeting* and ES cell technology. In addition, more recent refinements of this technology have led to the availability of conditional alleles that make it possible to alter gene function in a tissue- and time-specific manner (Lewandoski 2001; Anderson and Ingham 2003).

In this review I will focus on the developmental functions of an EGF-like signaling system, the Neuregulin/ErbB signaling system, which controls a multitude of essential processes during embryogenesis, as for example the development of the central and peripheral nervous systems and of the heart. Much of our knowledge about the biological functions of this pathway derives from the analysis of genetic models that have been established by the help of gene targeting in mice (Garratt et al. 2000a; Buonanno and Fischbach 2001; Citri et al. 2003; Falls 2003; Garratt et al. 2003; Holbro and Hynes 2004).

# 2
# Biology of the Neuregulin/ErbB Signaling Network

## 2.1
## Neuregulins and Their Receptors

Neuregulins (NRGs) comprise a large family of EGF-like signaling molecules that are involved in cell–cell communication during development as well as in the adult. They are primarily expressed in the nervous system, heart, mammary gland, intestine, and kidneys. Neuregulins transmit their signals to target cells by interacting with transmembrane tyrosine kinase receptors of the ErbB family. Receptor–ligand interaction activates intracellular signaling cascades that induce cellular responses including proliferation, migration, differentiation, and survival or apoptosis (Lemke 1996; Burden and Yarden 1997; Adlkofer and Lai 2000; Garratt et al. 2000a; Buonanno and Fischbach 2001; Yarden and Sliwkowski 2001; Citri et al. 2003; Falls 2003).

NRGs were first identified independently by several groups as factors that (1) activate ErbB2 (NDF, neu-differentiation factor; Holmes et al. 1992; Wen et al. 1992; Peles et al. 1993), that (2) stimulate Schwann cell proliferation (GGF, glial growth factor; Raff et al. 1978; Brockes et al. 1980; Lemke and Brockes 1984; Goodearl et al. 1993; Marchionni et al. 1993), or as factors that (3) induce acetylcholine receptors at neuromuscular junctions (ARIA, acetylcholine receptor inducing activity; Jessell et al. 1979; Falls et al. 1993). It turned out that the isolated proteins represent different isoforms encoded by the same gene, the NRG-1 gene (Falls 2003).

## 2.1.1
## The Ligands

NRGs are all characterized by the presence of an extracellular EGF-like domain (Fig. 1). The EGF domain alone is sufficient for activation of ErbB receptor tyrosine kinases. Alternative splicing gives rise to different variants of the EGF domain ($\alpha$ and $\beta$) that differ in their affinity to the receptor. By the use of distinct promoters, three major isoforms of the NRG1 gene are generated (Fig. 1): type I NRG-1 (neu differentiation factor, NDF; heregulin, HRG; acetylcholine receptor inducing activity, ARIA), type II (glial growth factor, GGF), and type III (sensory and motor-neuron-derived factor, SMDF; cysteine-rich domain neuregulin-1, CRD-NRG-1). The names first used in the literature for these isoforms do not typically reflect their major biological activities in vivo. For example, *glial growth* is primarily induced by type III NRG-1 in vivo, but not by type II NRG-1, (*glial growth factor*, GGF), which is, however, a potent mitogen for Schwann cells in vitro. The type I–III isoforms differ in the composition of their extracellular domains. Type I and II both have an Ig-like domain, which is located N-terminally to the EGF domain, and both isoforms are also referred to as *Ig-NRGs*. Type I NRG-1 possesses a glycosylated domain in addition. A cysteine-rich domain (CRD) is specifically found in type III NRG-1, and contains a hydrophobic anchor sequence, which results in a hairpin-shaped membrane topology of this isoform (Fig. 1). Both secreted and transmembrane NRGs are synthesized. Moreover, membrane-associated forms often contain internal proteolytic cleavage sites, and parts of the NRG molecules can be shed into the extra- or intracellular space (Bao et al. 2003). Interestingly, recent studies indicate that during evolution proteolytic cleavage of EGF-like ligands appears to be conserved but employs different classes of proteolytic enzymes: in mammals zinc-dependent, disintegrin-related, metalloproteinase-containing members of the ADAM family have been shown to cleave ErbB proligands. In contrast, in Drosophila, members of the rhomboid family of seven-pass transmembrane serine-proteases, which are insensitive to metalloproteinase inhibitors, can cleave membrane-associated precursors of the Drosophila homologues of TGFα (Urban et al. 2002; Seals and Courtneidge 2003). In a recent study Bao and coworkers provide evidence that interaction of type III NRG-1 with ErbB receptors allows *bi-directional* signaling, which involves proteolytic processing of the signaling partners as well (Fig. 8). First, ErbB receptors become phosphorylated upon ligand binding *(forward-signaling)*. Second, receptor binding to the ligand induces proteolytic cleavage of the ligands cytoplasmatic domain and its translocation to the nucleus *(back-signaling)*, where it represses pro-apoptotic genes (Bao et al. 2003). All NRG-1 isoforms show specific spatio-temporal expression patterns: type I NRG-1 is predominantly expressed during early embryogenesis, whereas type II is preferentially expressed in the nervous system during late development as well as postnatally. Type III NRG-1 is the major isoform expressed by axons of sensory and motor neurons (Meyer and Birchmeier 1994; Meyer et al. 1997).

More recently, additional NRG genes, NRG-2 (Don-1, NTAK), NRG-3, and NRG-4, encoding related proteins, have been identified (Fig. 1). They are encoded by different genes and partially differ in their expression from NRG-1 (Busfield et al. 1997; Carraway et al. 1997; Higashiyama et al. 1997; Zhang et al. 1997). Currently, much less is known about the functions of NRG-2, -3, and -4, in contrast to Neuregulin-1. Of the four NRG genes, NRG-1 and NRG-2 are the most closely related, and both possess two variants of the EGF-like domain, α and β, that differ in their receptor binding affinity (Jones et al. 1999). NRG-2 is expressed throughout the developing nervous system, and is also found in the embryonic heart, lung, and bladder (Busfield et al. 1997; Carraway et al. 1997). In the adult brain, NRG-2 expression is restricted to the cerebellum, dentate gyrus, and olfactory bulb (Busfield et al. 1997; Carraway et al. 1997; Chang et al. 1997). Postnatal expression of NRG-1 and -2 in the adult brain differs considerably, suggesting distinct biological functions in the adult brain for both genes. Interestingly, subcellular localization of NRG-1 and -2 on hippocampal neurons differs as well, for example, NRG-1 protein is targeted to axons, whereas NRG-2 protein has been demonstrated to colocalize with the dendrite-specific marker MAP2 in proximal dendrites (Longart et al. 2004; Talmage and Role 2004). Cell culture studies have further implicated NRG-2 in the activation of acetylcholine receptor (AchR) tran-

## Neuregulin Family

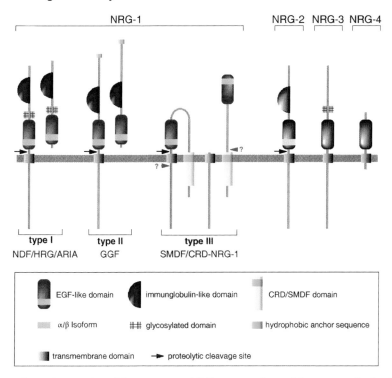

**Fig. 1** Schematic overview of the structure of different members of the Neuregulin family of signaling molecules. Neuregulin-1, -2, -3, -4 (NRG-1–4) are encoded by individual genes. All Neuregulins share an EGF-like extracellular domain. Alternative splicing of the C-terminal region of the EGF-like domain gives rise to $\alpha$ and $\beta$ isoforms, which differ in their affinity to the receptors. By the usage of different promoters various isoforms of the Neuregulin-1 gene are generated: type I (NDF, HRG, or ARIA), type II (GGF), and type III (SMDF, or CRD-NRG-1). Type I-III isoforms differ in the structure of their N-terminal, extracellular part. Type I and type II Neuregulin-1 both possess an Immunoglobulin-like (Ig) domain. A highly glycosylated domain, and a kringle domain (not shown) are located N-terminally to the EGF-like domain and are unique for type I, and type II Neuregulin-1, respectively. The type III isoform is characterized by cysteine-rich domain (CRD, or SMDF domain). This domain contains an internal hydrophobic anchor sequence, which allows this domain to take on a hairpin-shaped membrane topology. Proteolytic cleavage of the juxtamembrane domain generates a membrane-associated ligand in reverse orientation. Furthermore, proteolytic cleavage of the intracellular part of type III Neuregulin-1 can occur after binding of type III Neuregulin-1 to its specific receptor and has been implicated in reverse signaling. All Neuregulin-1 isoforms are synthesized as secreted or membrane associated forms. More-over, transmembrane precursor forms can be liberated by secondary cleavage. Neuregulin-2 is similar in its overall structure to the Ig-domain-containing isoforms of Neuregulin-1. No $\alpha/\beta$ isoforms have been identified for Neuregulin-3 and -4. Neuregulin-4 is the most distantly related Neuregulin molecule; in addition to its EGF-like domain Neuregulin-4 contains only a short cytoplasmic tail. For a detailed description see Sect. 2.1.1

scription, similar to NRG-1 (Rimer et al. 2004; Ponomareva et al. 2005). Unexpectedly, mice with a targeted deletion of the NRG-2 gene have been recently reported to be completely viable and do not display any overt mutant phenotype (Britto et al. 2004).

NRG-4 expression has been observed in the adult pancreas as well as in skeletal muscle and the central nervous system (Harari et al. 1999). NRG-4 can stimulate differentiation of somatostatin-producing cells in the endocrine pancreas in vitro (Huotari et al. 2002).

## 2.1.2
## ErbB Receptors

NRGs signal via tyrosine kinase receptors of the ErbB or epidermal growth factor receptor family. This family comprises four members, the epidermal growth factor receptor (EGFR, HER1), ErbB2 (Neu, HER2), ErbB3 (HER3), and ErbB4 (HER4). All members share structural similarities: ErbB receptors have an extracellular ligand-binding region, a single membrane-spanning region, and a cytoplasmic tyrosine-kinase-containing domain (Fig. 2). ErbB receptors are expressed in various tissues of epithelial, mesenchymal, and neuronal origin. Under physiological conditions, activation of ErbB receptors is controlled by the spatiotemporal expression of their specific ligands. Ligand binding induces the formation of homo- (for example ErbB1/ErbB1) and heterodimers (for example ErbB2/ErbB3), which in turn leads to the activation of the intrinsic kinase domain, resulting in the phosphorylation of specific tyrosine residues within the cytoplasmic tail (Fig. 2). By recruiting intracellular signaling molecules, like grb2, grb7, PLCγ, shc, or p85, to these phosphorylated docking sites distinct intracellular signaling cascades are initiated, which finally lead to specific cellular responses such as growth, survival, motility, and differentiation (Schlessinger 2000; Buonanno and Fischbach 2001; Yarden and Sliwkowski 2001; Citri et al. 2003; Falls 2003).

Affinity toward one or more ErbB receptors allows ErbB ligands to be subdivided into three groups: (1) EGF, TGFα, and amphiregulin, which bind specifically to ErbB1; (2) betacellulin, heparin-binding EGF (HB-EGF), and epiregulin, which serve as high-affinity ligands for ErbB1 as well as for ErbB4; and (3) neuregulins which can either bind with high affinity to ErbB3 or ErbB4 (Neuregulin-1 and -2), or to ErbB4 alone (Neuregulin-3 and -4). Two members of the ErbB receptor family have been previously shown to possess unique properties. First, ErbB3, despite its ability to bind Neuregulin-1 and -2 with high affinity, lacks tyrosine kinase activity (Guy et al. 1994). Second, ErbB2 is an orphan receptor and no ligand has been identified that binds directly to it and that directly induces receptor autophosphorylation. Several ligands, however, have been demonstrated in vitro to indirectly induce tyrosine-specific phosphorylation of ErbB2: Neuregulin-1 can bind with high affinity to ErbB3 and ErbB4 (Plowman et al. 1993; Carraway et al. 1994; Tzahar et al. 1994). This induces rapid phosphorylation of ErbB2 when both receptors, ErbB2 and ErbB3 or ErbB4, are coexpressed by the same cells (Peles et al.

## ErbB receptor family

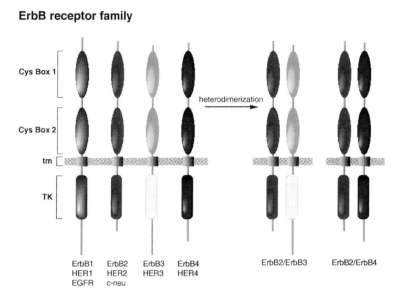

**Fig. 2** Schematic representation of the ErbB family of tyrosine kinase receptors. Shown are the epidermal growth factor receptor (EGFR, ErbB1, or HER1), as well as the Neuregulin-1 receptors ErbB2, ErbB3, and ErbB4. ErbB receptors are similar in their overall structure. All members of the ErbB family contain two cysteine-rich domains (CR1 and 2, or Cys Box1, 2) as well as two additional domains (L1 and L2) in their extracellular part, followed by a transmembrane (tm), and a juxtamembrane domain, an intracellular tyrosine kinase (tk) domain, and a regulatory region. Note that in contrast to the other family members ErbB3 has no active tyrosine kinase domain. Heterodimerization of receptor monomers gives rise to functional ErbB receptors, with ErbB2/ErbB3 heterodimers preferentially expressed in the developing peripheral nervous system, and ErbB2/ErbB4 heterodimers expressed in the heart and central nervous system

1993; Carraway and Cantley 1994; Sliwkowski et al. 1994; Wallasch et al. 1995). These in vitro observations suggested a central role for ErbB2 as an essential coreceptor for the transmission of the extracellular signal into the cell (Fig. 2).

### 2.1.3
### Receptor Activation

Recent elegant studies on the crystal structure of ErbB1, -2, and -3 receptors have provided important new insights into how ErbB receptor dimerization and signal transmission is regulated (Burgess et al. 2003). For many different ligand/receptor systems it is well established that receptor dimerization is achieved by the binding of a bivalent ligand to the extracellular domains of two receptor monomers, thereby crosslinking them into a dimer. This mode of action was first demonstrated for the human growth hormone and its receptor (deVos et al. 1992), and has been observed for several other receptor tyrosine kinases, like the vascular endothelial growth factor (VEGF) receptor Flt-1 (Wiesmann et al. 1997), the nerve growth factor (NGF) receptor TrkA (Wiesmann et al. 1999), and EphB2 (Himanen et al. 2001). Unexpectedly, the crystal structures of ligand-bound EGF receptor demonstrated that dimerization is entirely receptor mediated (Garrett et al. 2002; Ogiso et al. 2002). Contact between the receptor monomers is mediated by a prominent loop that extends from domain II (CR1) and has been named the dimerization arm (Ogiso et al. 2002). This domain II loop is specific to ErbB receptors, and mutational studies revealed that deletion of this region completely abolishes ligand-induced EGF receptor dimerization (Garrett et al. 2002; Ogiso et al. 2002). Additional interaction sites on domain II as well as on domain IV have been described. Yet their precise functional significance has not been determined (Burgess et al. 2003). Four distinct protein domains constitute the ErbB receptor extracellular regions, two homologous large (L) domains, and two cysteine-rich (CR) domains (Ward et al., 1995) organized in the order L1-CR1-L2-CR2 (or: I-II-III-IV). The relative orientation of these extracellular domains critically depends on whether a ligand is bound to the receptor or not. In the unbound, unactivated state direct intramolecular interactions between cysteine-rich domains II and IV occur. Interestingly, this interaction is stabilized through hydrogen bonds made by residues that are conserved in ErbB1, ErbB3, and ErbB4, but not in ErbB2. As a result, this domain II/IV tether buries the dimerization arm of domain II against domain IV and makes dimerization of the unactivated receptor in the tethered state impossible. Moreover, the ligand binding sites on domains I and III are kept apart from each other, hindering high-affinity ligand binding to the receptor in the tethered configuration. Yet, it is not clear, how a receptor is activated by its ligand. According to a current working model (Burgess et al. 2003) the presence of ligands is thought to shift the equilibrium between the unactivated (tethered) and rare activated (untethered) state towards the activated state. High-affinity ligand binding to domains I and III would thereby induce a dramatic conformational change, which leads to the release of the domain II/IV tether and in turn allows the dimerization arm to be exposed.

Moreover, crystal structure also helps to explain some of the unique biological properties of another member of the ErbB receptor family, ErbB2. Even without a ligand bound to the receptor, the extracellular region of ErbB2 resembles the activated form of other ErbBs with the dimerization arm constitutively exposed. Instead of the II/IV interdomain tether which normally covers the dimerization loop of an unliganded receptor, a close interaction between domains I and II occurs in ErbB2, which on the one hand appears to mimic interactions with a bound ligand, and on the other hand blocks binding of a ligand to the ErbB2 receptor molecule. In addition to the ligand-binding sites being obstructed in ErbB2 several residues expected to be important for ligand binding are mutated in ErbB2 (Cho et al. 2003; Garrett et al. 2003). Together these findings provide an explanation as to why no specific ligand for ErbB2 has ever been identified. Since ErbB2 is constitutively poised to dimerize, this may also explain the early observation that overexpression of ErbB2 can efficiently transform cells even in the absence of a ligand (for review see Yarden and Sliwkowski 2001). Furthermore, amplification or overexpression of the ErbB2 gene is found in many malignant tumors (see Sect. 2.4.1) and correlates with a poor prognosis. It appears controversial that biophysical studies failed to detect ErbB2 homodimers in solution or in crystals (Cho et al. 2003; Garrett et al. 2003). However, this may reflect a requirement that ErbB2 must be overexpressed at very high levels in order to transform cells, and that under physiological conditions ErbB2, because of its structure, may instead be ideally suited to serve as a heterodimerization partner for other members of the ErbB family (Burgess et al. 2003). Intriguingly, a role of ErbB2 as an essential core-ceptor for transmission of Neuregulin-1 signals was independently demonstrated in vivo by the help of mouse genetics. Comparative analyses of knockout mice with mutations of the ErbB2, -3, -4, as well as the Neuregulin-1 gene, unambiguously demonstrated that in vivo ErbB2/ErbB3 and ErbB2/ErbB4 heterodimers serve as functional receptors for Neuregulin-1 (for reviews see Lemke 1996; Adlkofer and Lai 2000; Garratt et al. 2000a; Olayioye et al. 2000; Buonanno and Fischbach 2001; Yarden and Sliwkowski 2001; Garratt et al. 2003).

Recent observations have added further complexity to the ErbB signaling model: Muc4 encodes a membrane-associated heterodimeric mucin that contains two epi-dermal growth factor (EGF)-like domains in its transmembrane region. Conserved residues within one of the EGF-like domains are similar to those within EGF do-mains known to activate ErbB receptors (Sheng et al. 1992). Cotransfection exper-iments in insect cells demonstrated specific binding of Muc4 to ErbB2, but not to other members of the ErbB family (Ramsauer et al. 2003). Moreover, Muc4 induces tyrosine-specific phosphorylation of ErbB2, even in the absence of ErbB receptor ligands. In the presence of Neuregulins Muc4 can potentiate receptor activation (Sheng et al. 1992). Interestingly, the activation profile of downstream targets of ErbB2 is different when Muc4 acts on ErbB2 alone, or when acting in concert with Neuregulins, suggesting a further level of receptor regulation. Thus, ErbB signal-ing is not only regulated by the types of Neuregulin ligands and the composition of receptor heteromers, but also by the simultaneous expression of additional, neighboring components capable of directly binding to ErbB2 (Carraway et al. 2003).

## 2.1.4
### Signal Processing

Specificity, duration and strength of ErbB-mediated intracellular signals are con-trolled by the ligand type, the composition of the receptor-dimer, as well as by the available spectrum of intracellular docking molecules that associate with specific phosphotyrosine residues on the cytoplasmic tail of an ErbB molecule. Which sites are phosphorylated, and hence which docking molecules are recruited to the receptors, is determined by the ligand and by the receptor heterodimer. Among the signaling cascades that are stimulated upon activation of ErbB receptors are MAPK, PI3 K, PLCγ, protein kinase C, and the Jak-STAT pathway. The Ras- and Shc-mediated activation of the MAPK pathway is common to all ErbB ligands, and the PI3K-activated Akt pathway is activated by most of the ErbBs. In addition, each receptor employs a specific set of signaling molecules: ErbB3 cannot bind c-Cbl, Grb2, PLCγ, or GAP, but can associate with Shc and Grb7. Within the nucleus such signaling events initiate transcriptional programs involving transcription factors like fos, Jun, and Myc, Sp1, Forkhead, as well as Ets family transcription factors (Yarden and Sliwkowski 2001). ErbB signals are turned off by mechanisms that depend on the receptor type and the composition of the receptor dimer. ErbB1 is the only receptor that is primarily targeted to lysosomal degradation whereas ErbB2, -3 and -4 are endocytosis impaired and are repeatedly recycled back to the cell surface. Moreover, ErbB2 decreases the rate of internalization while increasing the rate of recycling of its partners.

Still, our knowledge is limited about how distinct ErbB-dependent intracellular signaling pathways are able to elicit specific cellular responses, i.e., proliferation, migration, or survival. Very recently Nancy Hynes's group identified a novel intracellular signaling component, MEMO (*mediator* of *ErbB2-driven cell motility*), which specifically couples ErbB2 dependent signals to cell motility (Marone et al. 2004). MEMO most probably interacts with a phosphotyrosine at position 1227 through Shc. After ErbB2 activation, MEMO-defective cells fail to extend microtubules toward the cell cortex, indicating that MEMO controls cell migration by directly relaying ErbB2-mediated signals to the cytoskeleton (Marone et al. 2004).

## 2.1.5
### Crosstalk with Other Signaling Networks

ErbB receptors are not only the specific targets of EGF-like ligands, they also serve as integrators for signals emanating from heterologous signaling systems, thereby participating in a broader cellular signaling network (Gschwind et al. 2001; Prenzel et al. 2001; Holbro and Hynes 2004). Two distinct mechanisms of ErbB receptor transactivation have been described. First, ErbB receptors can serve as a scaffold that transmits information to downstream signaling pathways. This mode of interaction has been described for growth hormone (GH) and prolactin (Prl). Binding of these ligands to their specific receptors leads to the phosphorylation of the cytoplasmic part of ErbB1 or ErbB2 through the direct action of the tyrosine kinase Jak2, which is constitutively bound to the hormone receptors (Yamauchi et al. 1997; Yamauchi et al. 2000). In addition, the nonreceptor tyrosine kinase src is able to directly phosphorylate various residues on the ErbB1 receptor (Biscardi et al. 1999). In both cases ErbB receptors can interact passively, without any intrinsic kinase activity with neighboring signaling systems by providing docking sites for cytoplasmic downstream molecules, which may not participate in their own signaling pathways.

Second, ErbB receptors can be transactivated by another mechanism, which has been described as "triple-membrane-passing signal mechanism of EGFR transactivation," TMPS (Prenzel et al. 1999; Carpenter 2000; Prenzel et al. 2001). According to this model, G-protein coupled receptors (GPCR) and their specific ligands, like endothelin-1, thrombin, bombesin, or lysophosphatic acid (LPA) transactivate ErbB receptors through a rapid stimulation of cell-surface-associated metalloproteinases of the ADAM family, which leads in turn to the cleavage and activation of membrane-bound EGF-like proligands from the cell surface (Asakura et al. 2002; Yan et al. 2002; Seals and Courtneidge 2003). This process involves various intracellular signaling molecules, for example Src kinases, $Ca^{2+}$, and PKC. Released ligands can bind to and activate neighboring ErbB receptors, thereby linking GPCR-triggered signals to the ErbB signaling pathway. More recently, Wnt1 and Wnt5a signals have also been demonstrated to transactivate ErbB1 through a metalloproteinase-dependent release of ErbB1 ligands (Civenni et al. 2003).

## 2.2
## Developmental Functions of the Neuregulin-1/ErbB Signaling Pathway

### 2.2.1
### Neural Crest Cells and Their Derivatives

Neural crest cells constitute a pluripotent embryonic cell population that appears only transiently during development. Neural crest cells are defined by their origins at the lateral borders of the forming neural tube, by their stem-cell-like properties, and by their ability to migrate over long distances along invariant pathways through the embryo. After being specified in the dorsal neural tube epithelium, pre-migratory neural crest cells undergo an epithelio-mesenchymal transition. Such cells detach from the neural tube epithelium and start to colonize specific target sites within the embryo as undifferentiated, but not entirely uncommitted neural crest cells, where they give rise to all major components of the peripheral nervous system (Fig. 3), i.e., primary sensory neurons, multipolar neurons of the sympathetic and parasympathetic ganglia, enteric nervous system, Schwann cell glia along peripheral nerves, and satellite glia within peripheral ganglia, as well as cutaneous mechanoreceptors (Merkel cells). Furthermore, neural crest cells contribute to the formation of the cardiac outflow tract, to facial cartilage and bone, and to the melanocyte lineage (Anderson et al. 1997; Le Douarin and Kalcheim 1999; Halata et al. 2003; Szeder et al. 2003).

On a cellular level, development of neural crest cells and their derivatives involves processes like proliferation, survival, migration, and cell fate determination and differentiation. Neural crest development can be subdivided into three major phases: (1) specification of neural crest cell identity within the neural epithelium, (2) epithelio-mesenchymal transition, delamination, and directed migration of undifferentiated neural crest cells to their targets, and (3) target-site-specific differentiation into final cell types. Over the past fifteen years, key molecules in the control of neural crest cell development have been discovered (Anderson et al. 1997; Le Douarin and Kalcheim 1999; Meulemans and Bronner-Fraser 2004).

It has become clear from classical experimental studies carried out in different species, that signals from surrounding, nonneural tissues as well as cell-intrinsic

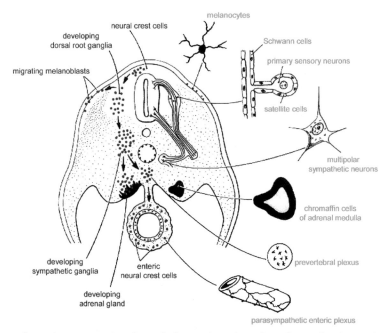

**Fig. 3** Schematic cross-section through the trunk region of a embryo, showing major sub-populations of developing neural crest cells and their characteristic migratory pathways (*left side, red*). On the *right side* (*green*) adult derivatives of the neural crest are represented. (Modified after Carlson, *Patten's Foundations of Embryology*, 6th edition 1996, McGraw–Hill, New York)

mechanisms are involved in the induction of neural crest cells at the dorso-lateral borders of the neural tube epithelium (Knecht and Bronner-Fraser 2002; Barembaum and Bronner-Fraser 2005). Nonneural ectoderm when juxtaposed to neural plate tissue can induce neural crest cells. Even nonaxial, lateral mesoderm, when cocultured with neural plates has been shown to elicit expression of some neural crest markers (Moury and Jacobson 1990; Selleck and Bronner-Fraser 1995; Marchant et al. 1998). Several recent studies have demonstrated inductive activity of these tissues to be conferred by signaling molecules of the Wnt, BMP, and FGF family. Probably the best experimental evidence for participation of extrinsic signals in this process comes from recent studies in chicken: addition of Wnt1-conditioned medium to naïve intermediate neural plate tissue is sufficient to induce the formation of neural crest cells in vitro (Garcia-Castro et al. 2002).

Furthermore, intermediate neural plates can give rise to neural crest in the absence of nonneural ectoderm, when BMPs have been added to the in vitro culture (Liem et al. 1995; Liem et al. 1997; Lee and Jessell 1999). Mice with a compound mutation of the Wnt1 and Wnt3a genes show defects in the early steps of neural crest formation as well, further supporting a critical role of this signaling pathway in this process (Ikeya et al. 1997). In addition to outside signals, several transcription factors have been demonstrated to control neural crest induction cell-autonomously. Sox9, a member of the SoxE subgroup of HMG-box containing transcription factors and the winged-helix transcription factor FoxD3 can both induce phenotypic properties of neural crest cells when overexpressed in the chicken neural tube, and loss-of-function analysis of Sox9 in Xenopus embryos further suggests that Sox9 is required for the generation of the cranial neural crest (Dottori et al. 2001; Kos et al. 2001; Spokony et al. 2002; Cheung and Briscoe 2003). Since neither factor is sufficient to promote efficient epithelio-mesenchymal transition and delamination of neural crest cells by itself when overexpressed in the neural tube, it has been speculated that both events are independently controlled (Dottori et al. 2001; Cheung and Briscoe 2003). Indeed, in a very recent, elegant study James Briscoe's group (NIMR, London) has shown that the coordinated activities of Sox9, FoxD3 and another zinc finger transcription factor, slug/snail, which was previously implicated in the control of neural crest cell migratory behavior (Nieto et al. 1994; LaBonne and Bronner-Fraser 2000; del Barrio and Nieto 2002), are required for the manifestation of all principal transcriptional and morphological characteristics of neural crest cells (Cheung et al. 2005).

### 2.2.1.1
### Sympathetic Nervous System Development

After detachment from the dorsal neural tube neural crest cells start to migrate away and follow defined stereotypic routes through the embryo where they finally reach their target sites. This suggests mechanisms are involved that (1) control the migratory capacity of neural crest cells and tell them when to go and when to stop, as well as (2) initiate repulsive and/or permissive signals to guide migrating neural crest cells along their way.

Neuregulin-1 is expressed at the origins as well as along the migratory pathways and at the target sites of trunk neural crest cells (Fig. 4; Meyer and Birchmeier 1994; Meyer et al. 1997; Britsch et al. 1998). Moreover, neural crest cells themselves express the receptor molecules ErbB2 and ErbB3, suggesting a paracrine signaling mechanism (Fig. 5; Britsch et al. 1998). Studies in mice with a targeted deletion of the Neuregulin-1 gene (Meyer and Birchmeier 1995) or its receptor ErbB2 (Lee et al. 1995; Britsch et al. 1998) have demonstrated that Neuregulin-1/ErbB signals directly control the migratory capacity of neural crest cells in the trunk (Fig. 5; Britsch et al. 1998). In homozygous mutant embryos, neural crest cells undergo epithelio-mesenchymal transition and detach from the neural epithelium but fail to migrate away from their sites of origin. As a consequence, only very few neural crest cells are detectable along the migratory routes and almost no cells ever reach their targets on both sides of the dorsal aorta. Instead, mutant neural crest cells stay close to their sites of birth, where they tend to form clusters (Fig. 5; Britsch et al. 1998). Both survival and proliferation of neural crest cells are not altered in the mutant animals, indicating that Neuregulin-1 signals directly control the migratory behavior of trunk neural crest cells. This migratory failure results in a severe

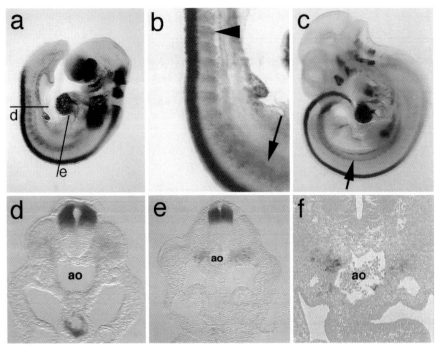

**Fig. 4a–f** Expression of type I Neuregulin-1 during migration of neural crest cells and the formation of the primary sympathetic nervous system. Whole-mount $\beta$-galactosidase staining of embryos heterozygous for the Neuregulin$^{lacZ}$ allele (Meyer and Birchmeier 1995) on E9 (**a, b**) and E10 (**c**); cross-sections of the embryo shown in **a** and **b** on a caudal (**d**) and upper forelimb level (**e**); cross-section of the E10 embryo shown in **c** on the forelimb level (**f**). *Lines* in **a** indicate the level of the section shown in **d** and **e**. The *arrowhead* in **b** points to somite-associated Neuregulin-1expression; *arrows* in **b** and **c** point to the mesenchyme-associated expression of Neuregulin-1 on both sides of the dorsal aorta (*ao*) (Picture reproduced by permission of Cold Spring Harbor Laboratory Press.)

hypoplasia of the primary derivatives of these cells, the primordial sympathetic ganglia (Britsch et al. 1998). Mice with a homozygous mutation of the Neuregulin-1 or the ErbB2 gene die around E10.5 due to defective heart development (Lee et al. 1995; Meyer and Birchmeier 1995; Britsch et al. 1998). Therefore, functions of this signaling pathway during later stages of neural crest cell development could not be analyzed in these mutants. However, ErbB3, which is the essential coreceptor of ErbB2 in neural crest cells, is not expressed in the myocardium and animals with a targeted mutation of the ErbB3 gene survive to birth albeit with reduced Mendelian rates (Riethmacher et al. 1997). Developmental defects of neural crest cells in ErbB3 mutant mice are indistinguishable from those observed in Neuregulin-1 or ErbB2 mutant mice, providing direct genetic evidence that neural crest cells receive Neuregulin-1 signals through ErbB2/ErbB3 heterodimeric receptors. Moreover, during later stages, ErbB3 mutant mice display a complete loss

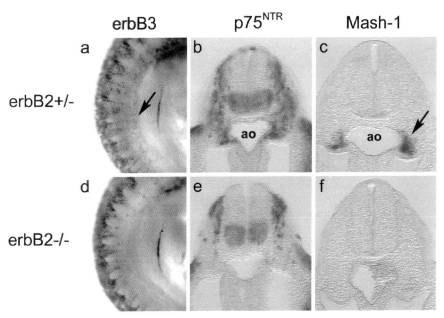

**Fig. 5a–f** Trunk neural crest cells require Neuregulin-1 signals for the maintenance of their migratory capacity. Migrating neural crest cells are visualized by in situ hybridization with riboprobes specific for ErbB3 (**a, d**), and the low-affinity neurotrophin receptor $p75^{NTR}$ (**b, e**). After neural crest cells have reached their targets on both sides of the dorsal aorta (*ao*) they undergo sympathetic neuronal differentiation, as indicated by the expression of the marker gene Mash-1 (**c**). Shown are lateral views (**a, d**) and cross-sections (**b, c, e, f**) of E9 mouse embryos heterozygous (**a–c**), or homozygous mutant (**d–f**) for the ErbB2 gene. In the homozygous mutant animals undifferentiated neural crest cells are generated from the dorsal neural tube, but fail to migrate along the characteristic pathways to their target sites (**d, e**; compare *arrow* in **a**). As a consequence, no Mash-1 expressing cells are detectable in these regions in homozygous mutants (**f**, compare *arrow* in **c**) (Picture reproduced by permission of Cold Spring Harbor Laboratory Press.)

of chromaffin cells of the adrenal medulla (Fig. 6) and a severe hypoplasia of para- and prevertebral sympathetic ganglia (Britsch et al. 1998). These structures are primary sites for the synthesis of catecholamines during development. Hence, levels of endogenous noradrenaline, which is the major catecholamine produced during embryogenesis, are approximately fifteen-fold reduced in homozygous mutant animals (Britsch et al. 1998). Tyrosine hydroxylase and dopamine-beta-hydroxylase are both key enzymes for the biosynthesis of catecholamines. Interestingly, mice with targeted deletions of these enzymes have been reported to die before birth with a similar time course of prenatal lethality as observed for ErbB3 mice (Thomas et al. 1995; Zhou et al. 1995; Riethmacher et al. 1997). This supports the idea that the prenatal loss of catecholamines in ErbB3 mutants is a major reason for embryonic lethality in these mice (Britsch et al. 1998).

## erbB3+/-          erbB3-/-

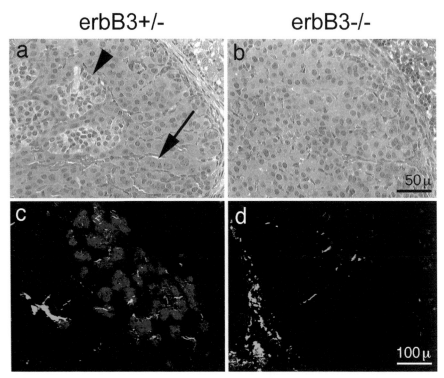

**Fig. 6a–d** Chromaffin cells of the adrenal medulla are absent in homozygous ErbB3 mutant animals. Appearance of the adrenal medulla in control (**a, c**) and ErbB3 mutant (**b, d**) embryos on E17.5. Histological sections were stained with hematoxylin/eosin (**a, b**); the *arrowhead* in **a** indicates islets of chromaffin cells within the adrenal gland. The *arrow* points to normal epithelial columns of the adrenal cortex. **c, d** Immunofluorescent staining of the adrenal medulla with antibodies directed against tyrosine hydroxylase (TH; *red*) and neurofilament (*green*). Note that TH-positive, chromaffin cells are undetectable in the mutant animals (**d**) (Picture reproduced by permission of Cold Spring Harbor Laboratory Press.)

Functions of Neuregulin-1 signals in the regulation of the migratory capacity of neural crest cells and their glial derivatives have been demonstrated in vitro as well: motility of neural crest cells is increased when cells migrate on stripes coated with neuregulin-1 ligand as compared to noncoated control stripes (Britsch and Birchmeier, unpublished data). Moreover, various groups reported neuregulin-1 to directly increase the motility of Schwann cells in vitro when added to the culture system (Mahanthappa et al. 1996; Meintanis et al. 2001). Correspondingly, the motility of Schwann cell precursors was found to be decreased in explants from mice with a null mutation of the erbB2 gene (Morris et al. 1999).

From these data one would expect prolonged neuregulin-1 signaling to result in an overshooting migratory behavior of neural crest cells or some of their derivatives. However, so far no activating mutations of components of the Neuregulin-1/ErbB2/3 pathway with such a phenotype have been described in the literature.

Expression of Neuregulin-1 and its corresponding receptors ErbB2 and ErbB3 are spatiotemporally tightly linked during migration of neural crest cells (compare Figs. 4 and 5). However, no guidance functions of Neuregulin-1 on migrating neural crest cells have been observed, indicating that additional factors may be required to help neural crest cells reach their correct targets. Along their way to the mesenchyme on both sides of the dorsal aorta trunk, neural crest cells migrate through the somitic tissues lateral to the neural tube. Interestingly, neural crest cell migration is restricted exclusively to the rostral halves of the somites. Wang and Anderson demonstrated different members of the Eph-family of transmembrane ligands to be expressed only in the dorsal half of the somite and to provide guidance information for neural crest cells while passing the somites (Krull et al. 1997; Wang and Anderson 1997). Eph family ligands and their receptors are well established in their ability to provide guidance information in various biological systems (Poliakov et al. 2004). Recently, semaphorins and their corresponding receptors, neuropilins, have been implicated in the guided migration of neural crest cells. Trunk neural crest cells express the receptor neuropilin2, while expression of its ligand semaphorin 3F is restricted to the dorsal half-somite. In mice with mutations of the semaphorin 3F or the neuropilin2 gene migrating neural crest cells lose their restricted segmental migration pattern and instead migrate uniformly through the somites. This demonstrates that repulsive semaphorin signals participate in restricting migration of trunk neural crest cells to their characteristic routes (Gammill and Bronner-Fraser 2002; Gammill et al. 2005).

Upon reaching their targets, additional extrinsic signals regulate site-specific differentiation of neural crest cells. The dorsal aorta, for example, has been shown to produce BMP-4 and -7, both of which induce sympathetic neuronal differentiation (Reissmann et al. 1996; Shah et al. 1996; Lee and Jessell 1999; Schneider et al. 1999; Howard et al. 2000).

### 2.2.1.2
### Schwann Cell Development

Neural crest cells also give rise to Schwann cells that line adult peripheral nerves. During development, Schwann cell precursor cells migrate along outgrowing spinal nerve axons where they further differentiate into myelinating and nonmyelinating Schwann cells, both surrounding accompanying axons (Jessen and Mirsky 2005). Neuregulin-1 signals are essential for regulating the migratory capacity of Schwann cell precursors as well. Accordingly, in mice with mutated Neuregulin-1 or ErbB2 genes pre-migratory Schwann cell progenitors are present near the dorsal root ganglia but fail to move away onto outgrowing spinal axons (Meyer and Birchmeier 1995; Britsch et al. 1998). Furthermore, the group of K.-F. Lee (Salk Institute, La Jolla) has used dorsal root ganglion explants from ErbB2 mutant embryos to establish an in vitro migration assay, and showed that migration of Schwann cell precursors is decreased in explants derived from ErbB2 mutants (Morris et al. 1999).

Mice with mutations of the Neuregulin-1 or ErbB2 gene die around E10.5 due to defective heart development. In order to circumvent this early embryonic lethality various, genetic approaches have been used that make an analysis of late developmental functions of the Neuregulin-1/ErbB2/3 pathway possible. First evidence for such functions came from the analysis of mice with a targeted mutation of the ErbB3 gene. Within neural crest cells and their glial derivatives, but not within the heart, ErbB3 serves as an essential coreceptor for ErbB2. Accordingly, developmental defects in neural crest cells and their glial derivatives are similar in ErbB3, ErbB2, and Neuregulin-1 mutants; heart development, however, is normal in ErbB3 mutants (Riethmacher et al. 1997). In an elegant genetic study, carried out in C. Birchmeier' group (MDC Berlin), defective heart development in ErbB2 mutants was rescued by re-introduction of the ErbB2 gene into the embryonic heart. This was achieved by expressing the ErbB2 cDNA under the control of the Nkx2.5 gene (*knock-in*) that is expressed in the embryonic heart (Woldeyesus et al. 1999). When crossing this allele into ErbB2 mutant mice, the resultant mice were mutant for the ErbB2 gene in every somatic tissue except the heart. Such mice survive to birth and allow analysis of peripheral nervous system development in the absence of Neuregulin-1/ErbB signals during late embryogenesis. In these mice, a near complete loss of Schwann cells occurs, and the remaining nerve bundles appear naked and defasciculated (Fig. 7). Corresponding phenotypes have been described in ErbB3 mutants, and in ErbB2 mutant mice, where cardiac functions of Neuregulin-1 signals have been rescued by heart-specific, transgenic ErbB2 expression, as well as in mice with a mutation of the CRD-rich isoform (type III, or SMDF isoform) of the Neuregulin-1 gene (Riethmacher et al. 1997; Morris et al. 1999; Wolpowitz et al. 2000). This isoform is expressed by axons of peripheral nerves, and serves as the major ligand for ErbB2/ErbB3 receptors on Schwann cells and their precursors (Meyer and Birchmeier 1994; Meyer et al. 1997). The loss of Schwann cells observed in Neuregulin-1 signaling mutants is not entirely attributable to functions of Neuregulin-1 signals in the control of Schwann cell precursor motility. Several in vitro and in vivo studies clearly indicate that

---

**Fig. 7a–i**  Lack of Schwann cells in rescued erbB2 mutant (erbB2$^{-/-}$R) and in erbB3 mutant embryos. **a–c** Whole-mount in situ hybridization of control (**a**), rescued erbB2 (**b**), and erbB3 mutant embryos at E12.5 with a Sox10-specific probe. Sox10-positive Schwann cell precursors observed along the cutaneous sensory nerves in controls (*arrow*) are absent in the mutants. Whole-mount in situ hybridization of E15.5 thoraco-abdominal walls from control (**d**), rescued erbB2 mutant (**e**), and erbB3 mutant (**f**) embryos with Sox10 as a probe; Sox10-positive Schwann cell precursors are observed that accompany thoracic nerves in the control, but are absent in the mutants. (**g, h**) Semithin sections through nerves of the brachial plexus of control (**g**), rescued erbB2 (**h**), and erbB3 (**i**) mutant embryos. The *arrowheads* in **g** and **i** point toward Schwann-cell-associated nuclei within nerve bundles. In mutant nerves nuclei are almost completely absent (Picture reproduced by permission of Cold Spring Harbor Laboratory Press.)

Neuregulin-1 signals regulate survival, proliferation, and differentiation of the Schwann cell lineage as well (Salzer et al. 1980; Dong et al. 1995; Grinspan et al. 1996; Syroid et al. 1996; Morris et al. 1999; Woldeyesus et al. 1999; Wolpowitz et al. 2000; Leimeroth et al. 2002).

## wildtype    erbB2-/- R    erbB3-/-

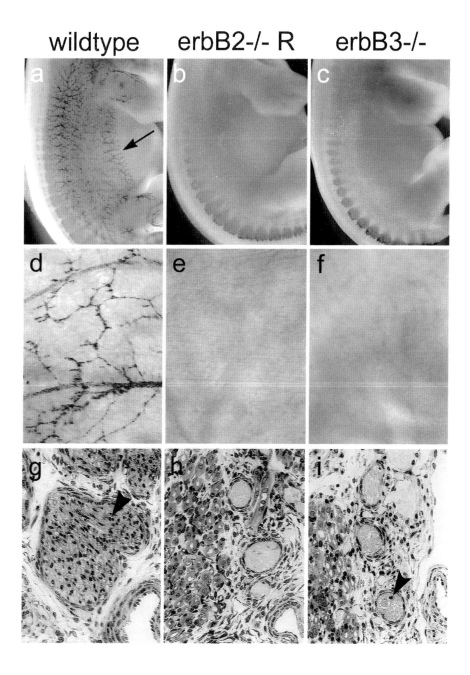

The zebrafish homologues of ErbB2 and ErbB3 have been recently identified in a genetic screen for myelin mutations (Lyons et al. 2005). Similar to the phenotypes observed in knockout mice, the most affected zebrafish mutants for the ErbB2 or ErbB3 gene lack Schwann cells throughout the entire peripheral nervous system (Lyons et al. 2005). By using a transgenic zebrafish line expressing green fluorescent protein (GFP) under the control of the FoxD3 promotor, migrating neural crest cells and their glial derivatives can be directly visualized in vivo. With this techniques Lyons and coworkers were able to directly demonstrate that in ErbB3 mutants, Schwann cell progenitors fail to migrate onto and along spinal axons. In addition, proliferation rates of GFP-expressing cells were reduced in ErbB3 mutant zebrafish embryos (Lyons et al. 2005). These observations provide striking evidence for conserved functions of ErbB3 in the development of the Schwann cell lineage in mice and fish (Lai 2005). Intriguingly, treatment of zebrafish with a pan-specific ErbB tyrosine kinase inhibitor causes reduced migration of FoxD3-GFP-positive cells. However, some cells remained axon-associated and motile. Such cells were frequently found to migrate retrogradely, toward the opposite direction, suggesting that ErbB dependent signals may provide directional cues as well (Lyons et al. 2005). This would be in line with a previous study in zebrafish that demonstrated peripheral axons to directly provide ErbB2/3-dependent instructive guidance cues for the migration of associated glia (Gilmour et al. 2002). It remains open whether this is a function solely mediated by Neuregulin-1/ErbB2/3, or whether more ErbB-receptor-involving signaling pathways are involved. In vitro data carried out on rat Schwann cells, however, support functions of the Neuregulin-1 pathway in directed migration of Schwann cell precursors (Mahanthappa et al. 1996).

During their development Schwann cell precursors proceed to become more differentiated, so-called immature Schwann cells (Lobsiger et al. 2002; Jessen and Mirsky 2005). This transition, which occurs in mice between E13 and E15, is accompanied by fundamental changes in the expression and response to survival signals and mitogens. Dependence on paracrine signals provided by axonally-presented type III Neuregulin-1 switches to autocrine signals provided by the Schwann cells themselves. Such signals include survival and/or proliferation factors such as insulin-like growth factor, NT3, PDGF-$\beta$, LIF, or LPA (Dowsing et al. 1999; Meier et al. 1999; Weiner and Chun 1999). Neuregulin-1 and its corresponding receptors ErbB2 and ErbB3, however, continue to be expressed by axons and on Schwann cells, respectively. In addition, Schwann cells, although becoming independent of Neuregulin-1, still respond to this factor (Chen et al. 1994; Corfas et al. 1995; Grinspan et al. 1996; Meier et al. 1999; Syroid et al. 1999). The analysis of mice with a Schwann-cell-specific conditional mutation of the ErbB2 gene first demonstrated in vivo that Neuregulin-1 has additional essential functions during late differentiation of Schwann cells (Garratt et al. 2000b). In these mice a widespread peripheral neuropathy develops with abnormally thin myelin sheaths and fewer myelin wraps (Garratt et al. 2000b). In a series of elegant experiments, the group of Klaus-Armin Nave (MPI Göttingen) recently confirmed that axonal Neuregulin-1 directly regulates myelin sheath thickness. Reduced Neuregulin-1 expression caused hypomyelination and decreased nerve conduction velocity, while transgenic overexpression of Neuregulin-1 type III in neurons under the control of the Thy1 promotor induced a dramatic hypermyelination. Interestingly, overexpression of Neuregulin-1 type I had no influence on myelination, indicating, that type III Neuregulin-1 is the critical component (Michailov et al. 2004).

During development, Schwann cells can adopt alternative axon ensheathment fates. Both are characterized anatomically as well as biochemically by the repertoire of proteins these cells express. Schwann cells can either associate with multiple unmyelinated small axons, forming a *Remak* bundle, or they can associate with an individual axon in a 1:1 ratio, and subsequently form a multilammelar myelin sheath around the axon. It is well established from classical experimental studies that this binary choice of axon ensheathment fates in Schwann cells is governed by axon-derived signals. In a very recent study, Neuregulin-1 type III was demonstrated to control this fate decision in Schwann cells (Taveggia et al. 2005). Ensheathed, nonmyelinated axons express low levels of type III Neuregulin-1, whereas myelinated fibers express high levels of the factor. The authors show that sensory neurons from mice deficient in type III Neuregulin-1 are defective in myelination. This defect could be rescued by lentiviral expression of type III Neuregulin-1. Moreover, overexpression of this factor converted sympathetic neurons, which are normally unmyelinated, into myelinated fibers (Taveggia et al. 2005).

Subsequent to their loss of Schwann cells, mice with a targeted mutation of the ErbB3 gene develop a severe degeneration of accompanying sensory and motor neurons. Similar phenotypes have been described in ErbB2 mutant mice with genetic rescue of ErbB2-dependent heart development and in Neuregulin-1 type III mutant mice (Riethmacher et al. 1997; Morris et al. 1999; Woldeyesus et al. 1999; Wolpowitz et al. 2000). Since ErbB2 and ErbB3 are not expressed by axons, neuronal degeneration has to be an indirect event that happens secondary to the loss of Schwann cells. In fact, chimeric analysis of ErbB3 mutants unambiguously demonstrated that neuronal degeneration occurs indirectly, i.e., in a non-cell-autonomous manner (Riethmacher et al. 1997): in mice that are mosaic for wildtype and homozygous ErbB3 mutant somatic cells, presence of little amounts of wildtype peripheral glial cells can rescue associated neurons from degeneration. This suggests that Neuregulin-1 type III interaction with ErbB2/3 receptors expressed by Schwann cells elicits Schwann-cell-derived signals required for the survival of Neuregulin-1-expressing neurons. Schwann cells have been previously shown to secrete several neurotrophic factors, like CNTF, BDNF, GDNF, LIF, PDGF, FGFs, IGF, and NT3 (Bunge 1993; Jessen and Mirsky 2002). However, in vivo evidence for direct functions in the survival of accompanying neurons remains poor. In a recent study, Corfas and coworkers have used dominant-negative ErbB expression to knock down ErbB signaling in adult, nonmyelinating Schwann cells. Mutant mice develop a progressive peripheral neuropathy with loss of unmyelinated axons and marked insensitivity to heat and pain (Chen et al. 2003). In these mutants, reduced glial-cell-line-derived neurotrophic factor (GDNF) expression was observed in affected nerves, and this may contribute to the degeneration of associated neurons (Chen et al. 2003).

Several observations have previously suggested that the Neuregulin-1/ErbB signaling pathway itself may allow bi-directional signaling and that transmembrane Neuregulin-1 isoforms can act as signal transducers in *reverse* direction as well:

1. Ectopic expression of Neuregulin-1 can induce apoptosis depending on the presence of the Neuregulin-1 intracellular domain (ICD; Grimm and Leder 1997; Grimm et al. 1998; Weinstein and Leder 2000).
2. Neuregulin-1-ICD can associate with intracellular signaling molecules like LIM kinase (Wang et al. 1998).
3. The intracellular domain of Neuregulin-1 type III is required for its function in vivo (Liu et al. 1998).

Talmage and coworkers demonstrated in vitro that type III Neuregulin-1 can indeed act as a bi-directional signaling molecule in neurons (Bao et al. 2003). Interaction of the type III Neuregulin-1 extracellular domain with ErbBs induces receptor dimerization and phosphorylation and the subsequent activation of downstream signaling events in the receptor-expressing cells (*forward* signaling). *Back* signaling, on the other hand, was shown to depend on binding of receptor dimers to the extracellular ligand domain and on neuronal depolarization. Receptor ligand interaction triggers the proteolytic release and translocation of the intracellular domain of type III Neuregulin-1 to the nucleus of Neuregulin-1 expressing neurons. Intranuclear Neuregulin-1-ICD in turn can suppress pro-apoptotic genes, which results in sustained neuronal survival (Bao et al. 2003). The significance in vivo of a *bi-directional* signaling mode for Neuregulin-1 type III remains to be determined (Fig. 8).

Interestingly, the extent and spatial distribution of motor neuron degeneration along the neuraxis follow a strict and characteristic pattern, with lumbar and cervical levels being most strongly affected (Fig. 9). This pattern of degeneration is identical in all Neuregulin-1 signaling mutants analyzed (Woldeyesus et al. 1999; Britsch et al. 2001). It indicates that motor neuron populations differ in their response to trophic signals, but the molecular mechanisms underlying these differences remain unknown. Molecular heterogeneity of spinal motor neurons, however, has been described, for example, in their expression profiles of different cadherins or LIM homeodomain transcription factors (Jessell 2000; Price et al. 2002). Furthermore, spinal motor neurons differ in their expression of the tyrosine kinase receptor c-met and their survival response to its specific ligand SF/HGF (Yamamoto et al. 1997).

Remarkably, neurological disorders in humans associated with motor neuron degeneration likewise often show characteristic patterns of neurons affected along the neuraxis. Hence, similar molecular mechanisms might be involved during development and disease of these structures (Suter and Scherer 2003).

Mice with targeted mutation of a specific gene are typically generated to determine selectively gene-specific functions in vivo. We have seen in the previous

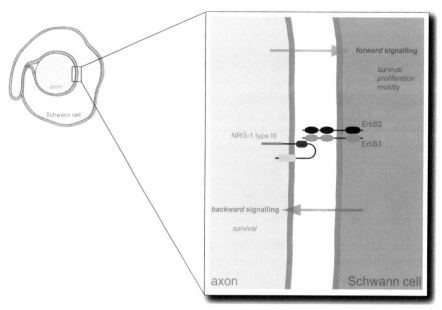

**Fig. 8** A model of bi-directional signaling by transmembrane Neuregulin-1 in peripheral axons and their corresponding Schwann cells. Both forward and back signaling result from interactions between ErbB2/3 receptor heterodimers and membrane-tethered type III Neuregulin-1. Ligand binding results in tyrosine kinase activation of ErbB receptors and subsequently induces cell survival and proliferation, and controls motility and differentiation in ErbB-expressing Schwann cells (forward signal). Interaction of ErbBs with the ligand further induces cleavage of type III Neuregulin-1 and the release of its intracellular domain (ICD). The released ICD can translocate from the axon membrane to the soma and to the nucleus of the neuron where it subsequently elicits biological events like neuronal survival

section that ErbB2 and ErbB3 mutant mice have also helped to uncover a critical role of Schwann cells in the maintenance of accompanying nerves, because such mutants entirely lack Schwann cells. This has allowed the assessment of peripheral nervous system development after selective ablation of this cell population (Riethmacher et al. 1997; Woldeyesus et al. 1999; Britsch et al. 2001). Similarly, using different strains of mutant mice, including ErbB3 mutants, as genetic tools, the lab of David Anderson (Caltech, Pasadena) has recently been able to resolve a longstanding question about the development of the embryonic vascular system (Mukouyama et al. 2002). During development small arteries and peripheral nerves of the skin develop in close vicinity and generate corresponding, complex branching patterns, raising the question whether pattern formation and differentiation of both structures are interdependent, self-organized, or may depend on extrinsic signals from other tissues (Martin and Lewis 1989; Shima and Mailhos 2000). In mouse homozygous mutants for the bHLH transcription factors Ngn-1 and -2 (Ma et al. 1999), that lack primary sensory neurons, cutaneous arteries

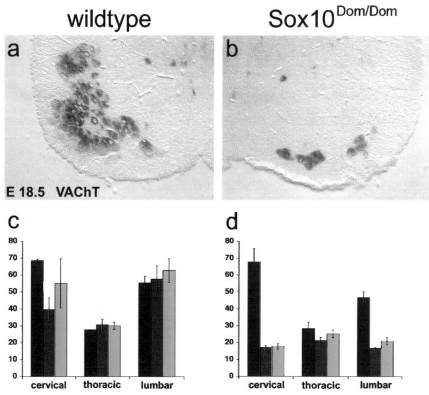

**Fig. 9a–d** Loss of motoneurons in Sox10$^{Dom/Dom}$ and ErbB3$^{-/-}$ mutant mice. Sections of the cervical spinal cord of wild-type (**a**) and Sox10$^{Dom/Dom}$ (**b**) mutant animals at E18.5 after in situ hybridization with a VAChT specific probe. **c, d** Motoneuron numbers in cervical, thoracic, and lumbar segments of spinal cords obtained from wild-type (*blue columns*), Sox10$^{Dom/Dom}$ (*red columns*), and ErbB3$^{-/-}$ (*green columns*) mutants at E15.5 (**c**) and E18.5 (**d**). Mean numbers of motoneurons per section +/– S.D. are shown (*n* = 4 embryos for each genotype and developmental stage) (Picture reproduced by permission of Cold Spring Harbor Laboratory Press.)

fail to differentiate properly and no remodeling of the early embryonic vascular pattern occurs (Mukouyama et al. 2002). Similar deficits have been detected in ErbB3 mutant mice at developmental stages where Schwann cells are lacking, but axons from sensory nerves are still present. Finally, in mice with a mutation of the axonal guidance molecule semaphorin 3A, an aberrant branching pattern of sensory nerves develops (Taniguchi et al. 1997; Kolodkin 1998), being adopted by the associated arteries. Together, these findings have provided direct genetic evidence that sensory nerves determine the differentiation and branching pattern of associated cutaneous arteries (Mukouyama et al. 2002). Furthermore, Schwann cells accompanying those nerves have been shown in vitro to act on associated blood vessels via the local secretion of VEGF (Mukouyama et al. 2002). This denotes a remarkable parallel to bi-directional signaling mechanisms at the interface of Schwann cells and accompanying axons. Since arterial vessels are known to produce neurotrophins (Scarisbrick et al. 1993; Francis et al. 1999; Donovan et al. 2000), the close association of blood vessels and sensory nerves may help the latter to recruit a local source of survival factors before they have reached their target sites (Mukouyama et al. 2002).

### 2.2.1.3
### Development of the Neuromuscular Junction

Once myoblasts fuse to form myotubes, they start to synthesize acetylcholine receptor (AChR) subunits that become assembled into functional receptors. Initially, AChRs are homogeneously distributed over the cell surface. With the innervation of the embryonic muscle, AChRs become clustered to membrane regions directly beneath a motor nerve terminal, where the neuromuscular junction (NMJ) forms. In the adult muscle AChRs are approx. 1,000-fold increased at neuromuscular synapses compared to extrasynaptic membrane regions. Although AChR clustering can occur spontaneously on cultured myoblasts, it is well established that motor axons are critical for the induction, maturation, and maintenance of the postsynaptic apparatus (Sanes and Lichtman 1999; Sanes and Lichtman 2001). The observation that inductive activity of motor neurons requires neither electrical activity nor transmitter release has led to the idea that motor neurons use chemical signals to organize the postsynaptic membrane. Several candidate molecules have been subsequently identified for their ability to increase AChR synthesis and/or clustering in vitro, among these is the acetylcholine receptor inducing activity (ARIA), which has turned out to be identical to Neuregulin-1 type I (Jessell et al. 1979; Falls et al. 1993). Since then muscle nicotinic acetylcholine receptor genes are probably the most extensively studied targets of Neuregulin function (Buonanno and Fischbach 2001). Developing muscles and cultured myotubes express ErB2, ErbB3, and ErbB4 receptors on their surface (Altiok et al. 1995; Moscoso et al. 1995; Zhu et al. 1995; Rimer et al. 1998; Trinidad et al. 2000). Like AChRs they localize to the neuromuscular junction by an agrin-dependent mechanism (Sanes and Lichtman 1999). Neuregulin-1 is expressed by motor neurons and secreted into the synaptic cleft. Neuregulin-1 signals have been shown to increase transcription of AChR genes in vitro and in vivo (Falls et al. 1993; Jo et al. 1995; Fischbach and Rosen 1997). Interestingly, adult mice heterozygous for a mutation-ablating Ig domain containing Neuregulins (i.e., type I and type II Neuregulin-1) are myasthenic and the density of postsynaptic AchRs is significantly reduced (Sandrock et al. 1997).

Mice with targeted deletions of the ErbB2, ErbB3, and the type III Neuregulin-1 have been employed to determine the development of the neuromuscular junction in the absence of Neuregulin-1 signals. All mutants show severe defects in the development of neuromuscular synapses with broadened, abnormally shaped synaptic regions, ultra-terminal sprouting of motor axon endings (Fig. 10) and reduced AChR expression in the synaptic region (Woldeyesus et al. 1999; Lin et al.

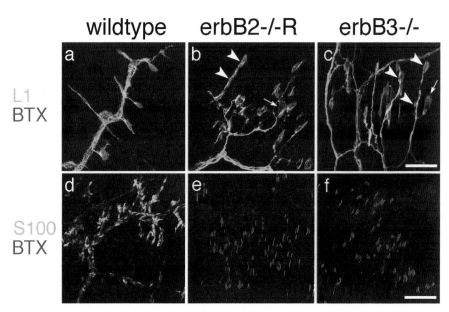

**Fig. 10a–f** Absence of terminal Schwann cells, and distribution of neuromuscular synapses in rescued erbB2 mutants and in erbB3 mutants. **a–c** Distal projections of thoracic nerves (11th intercostals nerves) and associated synapses at E18.5 were visualized with anti-L1 antibodies (*green*) and rhodamine-labeled a-bungarotoxin (*red*) in wild-type (**a**), rescued erbB2 (**b**), and erbB3 (**c**) mutant embryos. *Arrowheads* point toward multiple synapses associated with a single nerve branch, and *arrows* indicate large AChR clusters. **d–f** Schwann cells and terminal Schwann cells associated with distal projections of thoracic nerves and their synapses in control **d**, in rescued erbB2 **e**, and erbB3 **f** mutant embryos at E18.5. Anti-S100 antibodies (*green*) and labeled a-bungarotoxin (*red*) were used to visualize Schwann cells and clustered AChR at the synapse. Bars **a–c** 40 μm, **d–f** 100 μm (Picture reproduced by permission of Cold Spring Harbor Laboratory Press.)

2000; Wolpowitz et al. 2000; Yang et al. 2001). However, some AChR clustering and transcriptional specialization of synaptic nuclei occurred as well, indicating that Neuregulin-1 signals are not absolutely required for initial steps in the formation of the neuromuscular junction (Woldeyesus et al. 1999). The interpretation of these phenotypes remained ambiguous since all the mutants lack Schwann cells, even at the neuromuscular junction (Fig. 10) and the observed defects may reflect either direct or indirect effects of Neuregulin-1 signals. Furthermore, both ErbB2 and ErbB4 are expressed at the neuromuscular junctions and may have redundant functions (Rimer et al. 2004). To analyze neuromuscular synapse formation under conditions where Neuregulin signaling to the muscle is completely abolished, Escher and coworkers generated compound mutant mice with muscle-specific conditional deletions of the ErbB2 and ErbB4 genes (Escher et al. 2005). In these mice synapses form in skeletal muscles, clearly demonstrating that Neuregulin-1 signals to the muscle are dispensable for the formation and maintenance of the neuromuscular junction. Thus, effects of Neuregulin signals on the neuromuscular synapse are most likely indirect and mediated through peripheral glial cells (Escher et al. 2005).

Neuromuscular spindles (or muscle spindles) are mechanoreceptors that are essential for the control of muscle contraction. They provide proprioceptive information about the muscle tone and the position of the body in three-dimensional space. Each spindle contains a few small, specialized intrafusal muscle fibers, innervated by both sensory and motor nerves. This structure is surrounded by a spindle capsule of connective tissue. Similar to the formation of the neuromuscular junction, the development of muscle spindles critically depends on inductive signals from contacting neurons. Classical embryological studies have shown sensory but not motor innervation to be crucial for spindle development (Zelena 1994). Most proprioceptive neurons that provide sensory innervation of muscle spindles depend on TrkC-receptor-mediated neurotrophin 3 (NT3) signals for their survival. In mice with targeted deletions of the TrkC or the NT3 genes proprioceptive neurons are lost before their axons contact the muscle. Such mice lack muscle spindles (Ernfors et al. 1994; Klein et al. 1994). Interestingly, a defined population of proprioceptive primary sensory neurons from the nucleus tractus mesencephalicus develops independently from NT3 signals, however, in muscles innervated by these neurons muscle spindle differentiation is unaffected, indicating that NT3 itself has no influence on muscle spindle formation (Kucera et al. 1998; Matsuo et al. 2000).

Recent genetic studies have shown that the signal required for the induction of muscle spindles is provided by neuronally delivered Neuregulin-1 (Andrechek et al. 2002; Hippenmeyer et al. 2002). Conditional ablation of all three isoforms of Neuregulin-1 in sensory and motor neurons by an Islet-1-Cre mouse line abolishes muscle spindle differentiation and the expression of markers genes, selectively expressed by intrafusal muscle fibers (Tourtellotte and Milbrandt 1998; Arber et al. 2000; Hippenmeyer et al. 2002). Whereas most primary sensory neurons express the CRD-rich-domain-containing isoform of Neuregulin-1 (i.e., type III Neuregulin-1) in their axonal membrane, Ig-domain-containing isoforms (i.e., type I and II) are exclusively expressed by TrkC-positive proprioceptive neurons (Hippenmeyer et al. 2002). Conditional ablation of only the type III isoform in sensory neurons has no influence on muscle spindle formation, indicating that Ig-domain Neuregulins are essential for this process (Hippenmeyer et al. 2002). Furthermore, muscle-specific ablation of ErbB2 has been reported to result in spinal ataxia and the loss of muscle spindles (Andrechek et al. 2002).

It is characteristic of the Neuregulin-1/ErbB signaling system that a given developmental process is controlled by a specific ligand/receptor combination expressed by discrete cell populations. Sensory neurons, however, denote a remarkable exception, since they express different types of Neuregulins—type III and types I/II at the same time. Both are targeted to different cellular compartments, and act on different target tissues to control distinct developmental events: (1) type III Neuregulin-1 is targeted to the axon membrane and recognized by ErbB receptors on neighboring Schwann cells where it controls their differentiation; (2) type I/II

Neuregulins are targeted to the axon terminals and are recognized by neighboring muscle fibers where they control differentiation of the spindle apparatus.

## 2.2.2
## Central Nervous System Development

Neuregulin-1 and its receptors are broadly expressed in neurons and glial cells of the developing and adult central nervous system (Meyer et al. 1997; Buonanno and Fischbach 2001; Falls 2003; Anton et al. 2004). In contrast to the peripheral nervous system, terminal differentiation and maturation of the CNS occur late and extend far into postnatal life. As a consequence, a systematic in vivo analysis of Neuregulin-1 function in the central nervous system was limited by the embryonic or early postnatal lethality of the available mouse mutants. Much of our knowledge, therefore, is derived from in vitro studies. Further complexity of Neuregulin/ErbB functions in the central nervous system has been added to by the recent discovery of additional Neuregulin genes (Neuregulin-2 and -3). Both are expressed in the CNS and have been shown to activate ErbB4 (Zhang et al. 1997; Yarden and Sliwkowski 2001; Longart et al. 2004; Talmage and Role 2004).

Analogous to their essential functions in the development of Schwann cells, Neuregulin-1/ErbB signals have been implicated in the control of oligodendrocyte development (Barres and Raff 1999). In vitro, type II Neuregulin-1 (glial growth factor, GGF) promotes survival of oligodendrocytes and the proliferation of oligodendrocyte precursor cells purified from cortical cultures (Canoll et al. 1996; Fernandez et al. 2000; Calaora et al. 2001). GGF has also been reported to promote oligodendrocyte differentiation (Vartanian et al. 1994). In contrast, genetic studies failed to demonstrate unambiguously an essential function of Neuregulin-1 in oligodendrocyte development: in order to circumvent perinatal lethality Riethmacher and coworkers transplanted neural stem cells from ErbB3 mutant mice into the retina of newborn mice demonstrating that development of stem-cell-derived, ErbB3-deficient oligodendrocytes in vivo was normal (Schmucker et al. 2003). In addition, oligodendrocyte development is unaffected in adult ErbB4 mutant mice with cardiac rescue of ErbB4 function (Tidcombe et al. 2003). However, in a previous study, oligodendrocytes from in vitro cultured spinal cords of homozygous Neuregulin-1 mutant embryos failed to differentiate, and the oligodendrocyte-specific knock down of ErbB2 by the transgenic expression of a dominant-negative ErbB2 variant under the control of the MBP promoter has been reported to result in hypomyelination and apoptosis of oligodendrocyte progenitors (Vartanian et al. 1999; Kim et al. 2003b).

Based on their region-specific differential expression patterns, Neuregulins and their receptors have been proposed to control the composition and properties of neurotransmitter receptors on central neurons (Cannella et al. 1999; Steiner et al. 1999; Buonanno and Fischbach 2001; Ozaki 2001; Yau et al. 2003). In hippocampal neurons Neuregulin-1 can modulate expression and synaptic transmission of distinct types of GABA receptors in vitro (Rieff et al. 1999; Liu et al. 2001; Okada and

Corfas 2004). Neuregulin-beta, when added to slice cultures, induces the NR2C subunit of NMDA receptors on cerebellar granule cells (Ozaki et al. 1997). Yet, essential functions of the Neuregulin/ErbB pathway in the formation and biology of central synapses are still to be confirmed by gain- and loss-of-function studies in vivo.

During development, many neuron types of the brain utilize radial glial cells as a scaffold for their migration. Radial glial cells require Neuregulin-1 for their normal development, and these cells transmit Neuregulin-1 signals either by ErbB2 or ErbB4 receptors. Accordingly, disruption of ErbB2 has been shown to interfere indirectly with the radial migration of cortical projection neurons through the impaired development of corresponding radial glia (Schmid et al. 2003; Anton et al. 2004). In the cerebellum, Neuregulin-1 can induce astrocytes to take on a radial glial phenotype, which in turn supports migration of cerebellar granule cells in vitro (Rio et al. 1997). In addition to an indirect, *non-cell-autonomous* function of ErbB2 and ErbB4 in the radial migration of brain neurons, Oscar Marin's group (University of Alicante) has recently provided genetic evidence that ErbB4 exerts direct, *cell-autonomous* functions during neuronal migration in the brain (Flames et al. 2004). They showed a subpopulation of migrating interneurons derived from the medial ganglionic eminence (MGE) to express ErbB4. Along their migratory path to the cortex these neurons pass a tissue "corridor" that expresses a membrane-bound isoform of Neuregulin-1, whereas their cortical target sites express diffusible Neuregulin-1. Conditional ablation of either ErbB4 or Neuregulin-1 by the help of a forebrain-specific Cre mouse line (Hebert and McConnell 2000) perturbs migration of these interneurons to the cortex (Flames et al. 2004). This finally results in fewer GABAergic interneurons in the postnatal cortex. From their findings the authors suggested a model, according to which short- and long-range attractive and/or permissive signals, mediated by Neuregulin-1, control different steps of cortical interneuron migration (Flames et al. 2004; Flames and Marin 2005).

Neurogenesis in the adult brain is restricted to the hippocampus and the subventricular zone (SVZ) of the anterior lateral ventricles (Kornack and Rakic 2001; Alvarez-Buylla et al. 2002; Gage 2002). Neural progenitor cells from the subventricular zones migrate toward the olfactory bulb, destined to become olfactory interneurons. Interestingly, these progenitors migrate as chain-like structures without the guidance of radial glial cells, forming the so-called rostral migratory stream (Luskin 1993; Doetsch et al. 1997; Alvarez-Buylla et al. 2002). Neuroblasts in the subventricular zones as well as along the rostral migratory stream express ErbB4, and various Neuregulins (-1, -2, and -3) have been detected within this stream or in its close vicinity (Anton et al. 2004). The conditional disruption of ErbB4 results in defective migration and differentiation of neural progenitors toward and in the olfactory bulb (Anton et al. 2004).

Together, these findings not only underscore a general role of the Neuregulin/ErbB signaling pathway in the migratory control of forebrain neurons, they also draw an intriguing parallel to its functions in the control of cell migration during development of the peripheral nervous system.

## 2.2.3
## Heart Development

During embryonic development of the heart, Neuregulin-1 is expressed in endo-cardial cells, whereas its specific receptors, ErbB2 and ErbB4 are expressed by the adjacent myocardium, suggesting a paracrine signaling mechanism (Gassmann et al. 1995; Meyer and Birchmeier 1995). First evidence for a critical function of the Neuregulin-1/ErbB signaling system during heart development came from the analysis of Neuregulin-1, ErbB2, and ErbB4 null-mutant mice. These mice show corresponding defects in heart development, characterized by a lack of trabecu-lation, abnormally thinned myocardium, and enlarged heart cavities. As a conse-quence, homozygous mutant embryos die at midgestation, before E11 (Gassmann et al. 1995; Lee et al. 1995; Meyer and Birchmeier 1995; Kramer et al. 1996; Erick-son et al. 1997; Britsch et al. 1998; Liu et al. 1998). Elegant genetic approaches by several independent groups have unambiguously proven the essential function of Neuregulin-1 signals during embryonic heart development: in mice with a null mutation of the ErbB2 gene, a heart-specific function of ErbB2 was reconstituted by transgenic expression of an ErbB2 cDNA under the transcriptional control of heart-specific promoters (Nkx2.5, $\alpha$-myosin heavy chain promoter). In such animals with a heart-specific *rescue* of ErbB2 function cardiac development was normalized. Moreover, mutant mice with rescued heart development survived to birth, indicating that early embryonic lethality observed in null mutants is due to cardiac dysfunction (Morris et al. 1999; Woldeyesus et al. 1999). Several other mutations associated with similar defects in heart development have been de-scribed, for example, of the ShcA gene, which encodes an adaptor protein that transmits signals provided by ErbB and other tyrosine kinase receptors (Lai and Pawson 2000). Interestingly, a G-protein-coupled serotonin receptor (5HT-2B) is required for normal heart development as well. The mutation of the corresponding gene is embryonic lethal. Mutant animals lack trabeculae and have reduced ErbB2 levels in their myocardium (Nebigil et al. 2000). These data suggest a crosstalk between two discrete signaling pathways, and transactivation of ErbB receptors by G-protein-coupled receptors has been previously demonstrated for the EGF recep-tor (Daub et al. 1996). It is important to note that the demonstration of identical cardiac phenotypes in Neuregulin-1, ErbB2, and ErbB4 mutant mice has provided compelling genetic evidence that Neuregulin-1 signals are specifically transduced by ErbB2/ErbB4 receptor heterodimers in the heart. Accordingly, myocardial de-velopment, i.e., trabeculation, appears normal in ErbB3 mutant mice, since ErbB3 has not been reported to be expressed by the myocardium (Erickson et al. 1997; Riethmacher et al. 1997). However, additional studies have suggested functions of ErbB3 in the development of the heart valve mesenchyme and the heart cushions (Erickson et al. 1997; Camenisch et al. 2002).

Little is known about the molecular mechanisms underlying the process of trabeculation as well as the mechanisms by which Neuregulin-1 signals control this process. Trabeculation has been considered as a morphogenetic response of the myocardium (Lemke 1996). Mutation of a cardiac voltage-dependent sodium channel, SCN5a/Na$_v$1.5 also results in defective trabecule formation. SCN5a/Na$_v$1.5 has been implicated in excitation-contraction coupling. Thus, trabeculation may be also regulated by the physiological properties of the developing myocardium (Papadatos et al. 2002). Data from in vitro studies concerning cellular responses of cardiomyocytes to Neuregulin-1 signals are controversial (Garratt et al. 2003). However, some studies suggest Neuregulin-1 to be involved in the control of proliferation and survival of cardiomyocytes (Zhao et al. 1998; Baliga et al. 1999).

ErbB2 null-mutant mice with heart-specific reconstitution of ErbB2 function die immediately after birth, due to multiple developmental defects in the peripheral nervous system. Conditional mutation of the ErbB2 gene using the Cre-loxP system (Lewandoski 2001; Britsch 2006) has allowed the assessment of postnatal cardiac functions of the Neuregulin-1/ErbB pathway. Intriguingly, mice with heart-specific ablation of the ErbB2 gene survive into adulthood, but develop clinical and pathological features of a dilated cardiomyopathy with reduced contractility, secondary myofiber hypertrophy, thinned ventricular walls, and enlarged ventricular cavities (Crone et al. 2002; Ozcelik et al. 2002). It is currently unclear by which mechanism Neuregulin-1/ErbB signals maintain functional integrity of the adult heart. However, ErbB2 and ErbB4 expression has been detected in the T-tubule system where they could interact with components of the excitation-contraction coupling machinery (Ozcelik et al. 2002; Garratt et al. 2003; Ueda et al. 2005).

Because of potential clinical implications, the Neuregulin-1/ErbB signaling pathway in adult heart function has received great attention. This was very much accelerated by the clinical observation that treatment of breast cancer patients with a monoclonal antibody which specifically recognizes the human ErbB2/HER2 receptor (Trastuzumab, Herceptin) is accompanied by severe cardiotoxic side-effects, drawing a direct in vivo link from suppressed ErbB2 receptor signaling to impaired cardiac function (Slamon et al. 2001; Yarden and Sliwkowski 2001; Seidman et al. 2002). The role of ErbB2 mutants as models for cardiac diseases will be discussed in more detail in Sect. 2.4.1.

## 2.2.4
## Development of the Mammary Gland

Members of the EGF family of signaling molecules have been demonstrated to play critical roles during normal and neoplastic development of the mammary gland. For example, gene targeting experiments in mice revealed essential functions of the EGF-like ligands Amphiregulin, TGF$\alpha$, and of EGF itself in ductal differentiation and lactogenesis (Luetteke et al. 1999). Several lines of evidence have suggested functions of the Neuregulin signaling system as well: (1) Neuregulin-1 can stimulate lobulo-alveolar development and accumulation of secretory alveoli in mammary gland organ cultures (Yang et al. 1995); (2) exogenous Neuregulins, when administered to the mammary gland in vivo can induce proliferation and differentiation of ductal epithelia (Jones et al. 1996); (3) among the many existing

**Table 1** Synopsis of proposed functions of the Neuregulin-1/ErbB signaling system

| organ structure, cell type | function | *in vivo* | *in vitro* |
|---|---|:---:|:---:|
| **PNS** | | | |
| Schwann cells | Migration, survival, proliferation, of Schwann cell precursors, differentiation, myelination of Schwann cells | ✓ | ✓ |
| Sympathetic neurons | Migration of sympathogenic neural crest cells to target sites | ✓ | ✓ |
| Adrenal medulla | Migration of precursor cells to the anlage of the adrenal medullla | ✓ | |
| Muscel spindles | Induction, differentiation of muscle spindles | ✓ | |
| Enteric nervous system | Postnatal maintenance, survival of enteric neurons and glia[a] | ✓ | |
| Sensory/motor neurons | Survival of neurons, fasciculation of nerve fibres[a] | ✓ | |
| Cranial ganglia | Population of cranial sensory ganglia with neural crest cells | ✓ | |
| NMJ | acetylcholilne receptor synthesis and clustering | (Ø)[b] | ✓ |
| **CNS** | | | |
| Oligodendrocytes | Proliferation, survival, differentiation, myelination | Ø | ✓ |
| Cerebellar granule cells | migration along radial glia | | ✓ |
| Cortical interneurons | migration from MGE to cortex | ✓ | |
| Neural progenitors | Migration of neuroblasts along rostral migratory stream | ✓ | |
| Hippocampal neurons | Inhibition of LTP induction | | ✓ |
| Various neuron types | Regulation of GABA, NMDA receptor synthesis and function | | ✓ |
| **Heart** | | | |
| | Trabeculation of the embryonic myocardium | ✓ | |
| | Development of cardiac valves | ✓ | |
| | Development of the cardiac conduction system | | ✓ |
| | Maintenance of adult myocardial function | ✓ | |
| | Susceptibility to cardiotoxic drugs | ✓ | |
| **Mammary gland** | | | |
| | Epithelial proliferation, tubulo-alvolar differentiation during pregnancy, Lactation | ✓ | ✓ |

This list is not intended to be complete, it refers to the major subjects discussed in this review.

Abbreviations: PNS, peripheral nervous system; CNS, central nervous system; NMJ, neuromuscular junction; MGE, medial ganglionic eminence; in vivo, in vitro, experimental evidence based on in vivo, in vitro studies, respectively; Ø, function not observed in this type of study. For references see text.

[a] indirect functions of the NRG1/ErbB system;

[b] developmental defects of the NMJ observed in NRG1/ErbB2/ErbB3 mutants are most likely related to the lack of terminal Schwann cells in the immediate vicinity of synapses, and NMJ form when NRG signaling to the muscle is completely abolished (see text for discussion)

**Table 2** Overview of published mice with targeted deletions of components of the Neuregulin-1/ErbB signaling system

| Type of mutation | inactivated component | Developmental defects | | | timepoint/ cause of lethality | References |
|---|---|---|---|---|---|---|
| | | heart | PNS | mammary gland (during pregnancy) | | |
| **Ligands** | | | | | | |
| NRG1[-/-] | type I-III isoforms | + | + | n.a. | E10.5 (heart) | (Erickson et al. 1997; Meyer and Birchmeier, 1995) |
| CRD-NRG1[-/-] | type III isoform | normal | + | n.a. | birth (PNS) | (Wolpowitz et al. 2000) |
| Ig-NRG1[-/-] | type I and II | + | normal[a] | n.a. | E10.5 (heart) | (Kramer et al. 1996) |
| CT-NRG1[-/-] | cytoplasmic tail, type I (II, III?) | + | n.d. | n.a. | E10.5 (heart) | (Liu et al. 1998) |
| NRG1α[-/-] | α-isoform of EFG-like domain | normal | normal | + | normal lifespan | (Li et al. 2002) |
| NRG1[flox/flox] | conditional, NRG1 | | | | depending on Cre activity[c] | |
| **Receptors** | | | | | | |
| erbB2[-/-] | ErbB2 | + | + | n.a. | E10.5 (heart) | (Britsch et al. 1998; Erickson et al. 1997; Lee et al. 1995) |
| erbB3[-/-] | ErbB3 | Normal[b] | + | n.a. | birth (PNS) | (Erickson et al. 1997; Riethmacher et al. 1997) |
| erbB4[-/-] | ErbB4 | + | normal | n.a. | E10.5 (heart) | (Gassmann et al. 1995) |
| erbB2[-/-]R | ErbB2 in all tissues except heart | normal | + | n.a. | birth (PNS) | (Morris et al. 1999; Woldeyesus et al. 1999) |
| erbB4[-/-]R | ErbB4 in all tissues except heart | normal | normal | + | normal lifespan | (Tidcombe et al. 2003) |
| erbB2[flox/flox] | conditional, ErbB2 | | | | depending on Cre activity[c] | |
| erbB4[flox/flox] | conditional, ErbB4 | | | | depending on Cre activity[c] | |

Abbreviations: n.a., not accessible to analysis because of early lethality of mutant mice; n.d., not determined; +, developmental defects observed in the corresponding organ system (see text for detailed description).

[a] except the development of muscle spindles, which requires Ig-domain NRGs. [b] trabeculation of the myocardium occurs normal in erbB3[-/-] mice, deficits in the development of valves have been reported in one study (Erickson et al. 1997), but have not been confirmed by others. [c] see text for detailed discussion of studies using conditional mutagenesis of NRG1, erbB2 and erbB4 in mice

isoforms of the Neuregulin-1 gene only one particular isoform, the $\alpha$ isoform, is expressed by breast tissue and its dynamic expression correlates with epithelial differentiation (Yang et al. 1995); finally, (4) a dual function of Neuregulins in epithelial proliferation and differentiation has been extensively described in vitro in various mammary tumor cell lines, as well as in normal mammary epithelial cells (Li et al. 2002). Due to the embryonic or early postnatal lethality of many Neuregulin-1/ErbB signaling mutants, rigorous assessment of the precise roles of Neuregulin-1 during breast development in vivo has remained elusive until a selective mouse mutant of Neuregulin-1$\alpha$ became available (Li et al. 2002). Since this isoform is not involved in development of the embryonic heart or peripheral nervous system, homozygous Neuregulin-1$\alpha$ mutant mice survive into adulthood and can be used to analyze postnatal mammary gland development. In these mice epithelial proliferation and tubulo-alveolar differentiation were impaired during pregnancy. Moreover, mutant mice failed to express genes associated with the normal milk production (Li et al. 2002). Mice with conditional ablation of the ErbB4 gene in the developing mammary gland, and ErbB4 null mice with cardiac rescue of ErbB4 function display similar defects in mammary epithelial differentiation as described for the Neuregulin-1$\alpha$ mutation (Long et al. 2003; Tidcombe et al. 2003). Altogether, these observations indicate that Neuregulin-1/ErbB4 signals are essential for normal terminal differentiation and lactation of the postnatal mammary gland.

During embryogenesis, specification of the mammary gland epithelium is induced by mesenchyme-derived signals. Interestingly, in a very recent publication another member of the Neuregulin family has been implicated in the regulation of this developmental event. In a naturally occurring mouse mutant, *scaramanga* (*ska*), specification of the mammary epithelium is impaired (Howard and Gusterson 2000a; Howard and Gusterson 2000b). Positional cloning identified the Neuregulin-3 gene to be mutated in *ska* mice (Howard et al. 2005). Neuregulin-3 is expressed by the mesenchyme surrounding the presumptive mammary regions prior to the morphological appearance of a mammary gland primordium or the expression of specific epithelial differentiation markers (Zhang et al. 1997; Howard et al. 2005). A function of Neuregulin-3 as a paracrine, mesenchyme-derived signal is supported by its ability to directly induce mammary bud formation in explant cultures (Howard et al. 2005). Thus, different members of the Neuregulin family appear to control sequentially discrete steps during pre- and postnatal development of the mammary gland epithelium.

Neuregulin-3 has been previously demonstrated to bind to and activate ErbB4 receptors (Zhang et al. 1997). The apparent discrepancy, however, between the phenotypes in Neuregulin-3 and ErbB4 mutant mice—early specification of the mammary epithelium occurs normally in ErbB4 mutant mice—suggests additional ErbB receptors to be involved in the transmission of Neuregulin-3 signals in the mammary gland.

## 2.3
## Interacting Molecules—the Sox10/ErbB3 Connection

Until recently, available data relating to molecules that act upstream of components of the Neuregulin-1/ErbB signaling pathway were limited (Buonanno and
Fischbach 2001; Yarden and Sliwkowski 2001; Citri et al. 2003; Falls 2003). The
SRY-box transcription factor Sox10 was the first molecule to be identified that
controls the expression of the Neuregulin-1 receptor ErbB3 in a cell-type-specific
manner (Britsch et al. 2001).

Sox genes encode a group of proteins that carry a highly conserved SRY-box
DNA-binding domain, and additional domains implicated in transcriptional regulation (Kamachi et al. 2000). To date, more than twenty Sox genes and their
corresponding proteins have been identified. Members of the Sox family are clas-
sified according to sequence similarities within their SRY-box as well as to their
functions as transcriptional repressors, or activators. Sox genes are expressed by
various tissues in a cell-type-specific manner and have been demonstrated to be
key players in the regulation of embryonic development and cell fate determination
(Pevny and Lovell-Badge 1997; Wegner 1999; Kamachi et al. 2000; Hong and Saint-
Jeannet 2005; Wegner and Stolt 2005). Typically, Sox proteins are multifunctional,
either controlling independent developmental processes during embryogenesis, or
exerting sequential functions within the same developmental system. For example,
Sox9 controls developmental events as diverse as sex determination, chondrogen-
esis, or cell-type specification in the neural tube, while also being required during
sequential steps of chondrocyte differentiation (Akiyama et al. 2002; Wilson and
Koopman 2002; Stolt et al. 2003; Lefebvre and Smits 2005). Other Sox genes have
been shown to be essential for the development of the nervous system, for lym-
phopoesis, and lens development (Wegner 1999).

Sox10 was first identified in a PCR-based screen for novel SRY-like HMG-box
genes by Michael Wegner's group at the University of Erlangen (Kuhlbrodt et al.
1998a; Wegner 1999). Sox10 acts as a transcriptional activator and, together with
Sox9, belongs to the group E of Sox family members (Wegner 1999; Kamachi et al.
2000). Sox10 is expressed by undifferentiated neural crest cells immediately after
their generation from the dorsal neural tube and expression is maintained in those
cells that undergo glial or melanocytic differentiation (Fig. 11; Herbarth et al. 1998;
Kuhlbrodt et al. 1998a; Pusch et al. 1998; Britsch et al. 2001; Kim et al. 2003a). In
addition, Sox10 expression has been reported in the enteric nervous system, as
well as in oligodendrocytes of the central nervous system.

In the Jackson Laboratories in 1984, a spontaneous mouse mutation arose
named *Dom*. Mice heterozygous for the *Dom* allele are characterized by a white
belly spot, and the absence of enteric ganglia within the distal colon, leading to
a variable megacolon (*Dom* = dominant megacolon). In the homozygous state
the *Dom* mutation was found to be embryonic lethal, and a portion of heterozygous *Dom* mutant mice die within the first weeks after birth (Lane and
Liu 1984).

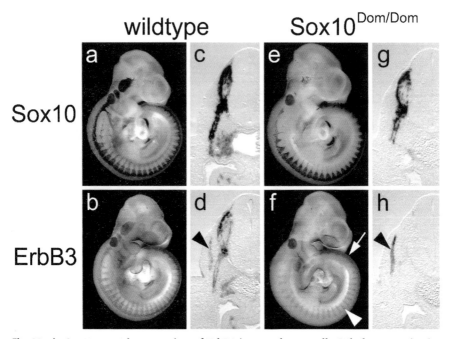

**Fig. 11a–h** Sox10 controls expression of ErbB3 in neural crest cells. Whole-mount in situ hybridizations of wild-type (a–d) and Sox10$^{Dom/Dom}$ (e–h) embryos with probes specific for Sox10 (*top*), and ErbB3 (*bottom*). Shown are lateral (**a, b, e, f**) views of E10.5 embryos and the corresponding vibratome sections (**c, d, g, h**) on forelimb levels. *Arrowheads* in **d, f**, and **h** point toward the myotome that also expresses ErbB3. Note that newly generated neural crest cells transiently express ErbB3 independent of Sox10 function (*arrow* in **f**) (Picture reproduced by permission of Cold Spring Harbor Laboratory Press.)

Bill Pavan's group at the NIH, and Michael Wegner's at the ZMNHamburg independently demonstrated the Sox10 gene to be mutated in *Dom* mice. A point mutation in the open reading frame of the Sox10 gene leads to a frame shift, and the generation of a premature termination signal. From the mutant locus, stable transcripts are generated that encode a truncated, nonfunctional Sox10 protein, with a deleted transactivation domain (Fig. 12; Herbarth et al. 1998; Southard-Smith et al. 1998).

### 2.3.1
### ErbB3-Dependent Functions of Sox10

A systematic analysis of the expression of ErbB3 and Sox10 during embryonic development revealed both genes to be expressed in almost identical spatiotemporal patterns (Britsch et al. 2001). Both genes are expressed in neural crest cells immediately after their birth from the neuroepithelium of the dorsal neural tube. Coexpression of Sox10 and ErbB3 is sustained in primary derivatives of the neural crest, like dorsal root and cranial ganglia anlagen, the primordial sympathetic

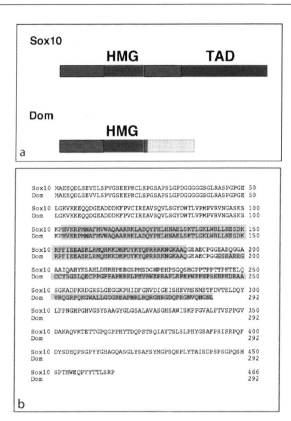

**Fig. 12a,b** a Schematic representation of the domain organization of wildtype Sox10 and the Sox10$^{Dom}$ protein (*HMG*, HMG-box DNA binding domain; *TAD*, transactivation domain). **b** Amino acid sequences derived from the Sox10 wildtype allele and from the Sox10$^{Dom}$ allele. In the Sox10$^{Dom}$ allele a point mutation results in a frameshift at aa position 194 and the generation of a truncated protein, which lacks its transactivation domain. HMG-box and truncated part of the mutant protein are highlighted in *red* and *green*, respectively

nervous system, and vagal neural crest cells, which enter the primitive intestine and contribute to the developing enteric nervous system (Fig. 11). Both genes, however, possess nonoverlapping expression domains. ErbB3 but not Sox10 is expressed in the myotome, whereas Sox10 but not ErbB3 is expressed in the melanocytic lineage (Britsch et al. 2001). Together, these findings suggested that both genes interact genetically. Analysis of Sox10 and ErbB3 expression in homozygous ErbB3 and *Dom* mutant mice, respectively, demonstrated that ErbB3 expression in neural crest cells depends on Sox10 function (Britsch et al. 2001). In homozygous *Dom* mutants, no ErbB3 gene expression is detectable in migrating trunk neural crest cells nor in those crest cells that have colonized their primary targets on both sides of the neural tube, the dorsal aorta, or along outgrowing spinal nerves (Fig. 11). The ErbB3 gene is transiently expressed independently of

Sox10 in newly generated neural crest cells during earlier developmental stages, but these cells require Sox10 function to maintain ErbB3 gene expression immediately after they have started to migrate away from their origins (Britsch et al. 2001). This is supported by the in vitro observation that Sox10 can increase ErbB3 expression in N2A cells (Britsch et al. 2001). It is unclear whether the interaction of Sox10 and the ErbB3 gene is direct or indirect, and no Sox10 responsive element has been identified in the genomic locus of ErbB3. However, the rapid induction of ErbB3 by Sox10 in cell culture argues in favor of a direct interaction. Recent experimental data have shown that individual HMG domains of Sox proteins are similar to each other in their sequence preference and DNA binding activity, indicating that binding to a specific target must be determined by additional mechanisms, as for example flanking DNA sequences, and multiprotein complexes (Kamachi et al. 2000; Mollaaghababa and Pavan 2003). In the case of the $P_0$ gene, which encodes a myelin-associated glycoprotein, and which has been shown to be a direct Sox10 target, flanking DNA sequences and the binding of Sox10 as a dimer are critical for the interaction of Sox10 with its specific target (Peirano et al. 2000; Peirano and Wegner 2000). The tyrosine kinase receptor c-ret is essential for the survival of neural crest cells that enter the intestine and contribute to the development of the enteric nervous system (Schuchardt et al. 1994; Schuchardt et al. 1995; Durbec et al. 1996). Mice with mutations of both the Sox10 and the c-ret gene develop a megacolon due to the apoptotic loss of enteric ganglia (Schuchardt et al. 1994; Durbec et al. 1996; Herbarth et al. 1998; Southard-Smith et al. 1998; Kapur 1999; Southard-Smith et al. 1999). Intriguingly, Sox10 has been shown to control expression of c-ret in enteric neural crest cells by direct protein-protein interaction with an additional transcription factor, Pax3, that binds to the c-ret gene in the close vicinity of the Sox10 binding site (Lang et al. 2000; Lang and Epstein 2003). The requirement of a partner factor in order to exert transcriptional regulation of a given target gene has been demonstrated for several other Sox proteins (Kamachi et al. 2000). It is tempting to speculate that in the case of the regulation of ErbB3 expression by Sox10, additional proteins, yet to be determined, are also involved.

Since Sox10 mutant animals lack ErbB3 expression in neural crest cells, both Sox10 and ErbB3 mutant mice show very similar defects in neural crest cell development. Both mutants have an impaired development of cranial ganglia, a severe hypoplasia of the trunk sympathetic nervous system, and reduced numbers of Schwann cell precursors along outgrowing spinal nerves (Erickson et al. 1997; Riethmacher et al. 1997; Britsch et al. 1998; Britsch et al. 2001). Interestingly, migration of neural crest cells has been described to be less severely affected in Sox10 mutants, which is most likely due to the short period of expression of ErbB3 independently of Sox10 function in newly generated neural crest cells (Britsch et al. 2001).

In addition to ErbB3-dependent developmental functions of Sox10, this transcription factor has been shown to execute ErbB3-independent developmental functions. In homozygous *Dom* mutants, development of the enteric nervous system and of the melanocytic lineage are severely affected; however, their development is unaffected in ErbB3 mutant mice.

Moreover, Sox10 has been demonstrated to play an ErbB3-independent key role in the development of the peripheral glial cell lineage (Britsch et al. 2001).

## 2.3.2
## Sox10 and Glial Cell Development

Neuregulin-1/ErbB2/ErbB3 signals are essential for Schwann cell development. Genetic ablation of this signaling pathway results in the complete loss of Schwann cells within the entire peripheral nervous system (see also Sect. 2.2.1.2). However, the expression of specific marker genes, like Notch-1 or B-FABP (Weinmaster et al. 1991; Kurtz et al. 1994; Meier et al. 1999; Morris et al. 1999; Jessen and Mirsky 2002), in differentiating glial precursors along spinal nerves or within dorsal root ganglia, is still detectable at E11.5, indicating that neural crest cells are able to take on a glial cell fate in the absence of Neuregulin-1 signals (Fig. 13). Nonetheless, Neuregulin-1 signals are indispensable for the migration, survival, and proliferation of Schwann cells and their precursors (Meyer and Birchmeier 1995; Riethmacher et al. 1997; Woldeyesus et al. 1999; Wolpowitz et al. 2000; Britsch et al. 2001). Sox10 also controls ErbB3 expression in Schwann cells, and expression of both genes is sustained in the peripheral glial lineage during further development. Therefore, Sox10 mutants were initially expected to have defects in peripheral glial development similar to those of Neuregulin-1 signaling mutants. Surprisingly, undifferentiated neural crest cells completely fail to acquire a glial fate in Sox10 mutants (Fig. 13; Britsch et al. 2001; Sonnenberg-Riethmacher et al. 2001). Despite this, neural crest cells expressing Sox10 from the mutant locus are still detectable at the sites where they normally differentiate into satellite and Schwann cell glia (Britsch et al. 2001; Sonnenberg-Riethmacher et al. 2001). These cells retain their undifferentiated state, and fail to take on alternative differentiation fates, and during the subsequent development are eliminated by apoptosis (Britsch et al. 2001). A critical role for Sox10 in glial differentiation from undifferentiated neural crest cells has been confirmed by in vitro studies (Paratore et al. 2001). Furthermore, overexpression of Sox10 in undifferentiated neural crest cells in vitro results in retention of their stem-cell-like properties and their capacity to acquire different cell fates (Kim et al. 2003a).

The precise molecular mechanisms underlying the determination of a glial fate and the differentiation of the glial cell lineage in the peripheral nervous system are still incompletely understood; Sox10 was the first molecule demonstrated in vivo to possess a key function in these processes. Expression of the Notch-1 receptor or its intracellular effector Hes-5 in neural crest cells is lost in homozygous Sox10 mutant mice (Britsch et al. 2001). The Delta/Notch signaling pathway is well established to control various cell fate determination events in the developing nervous system (Artavanis-Tsakonas et al. 1999; Baker 2000; Wang and Barres 2000). Interestingly, it was recently shown in vitro that transient activation of the Delta/Notch pathway in neural crest cells irreversibly induces glial differentiation at the expense of a neuronal fate (Morrison et al. 2000; Wakamatsu et al. 2000). It remains to be

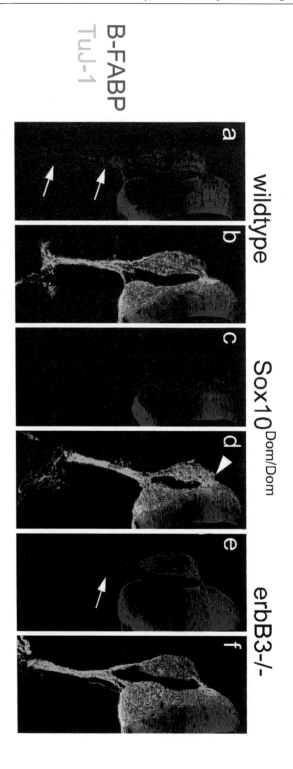

◀——————————————————————————————————————————————

**Fig. 13a–f** Sox10 controls peripheral glial cell development. Immunohistological analysis of wild-type (**a**, **b**), Sox10$^{Dom/Dom}$ (**c**, **d**), and ErbB3$^{-/-}$ (**e**, **f**) embryos at E11.5 on lumbar axial levels, using antibodies against B-FABP (*red*) and TuJ-1(*green*) to visualize peripheral glial cells and neuronal cells, respectively. B-FABP antibody signals (**a**, **c**, **e**) and an overlay of B-FABP and TuJ-1 antibody signals (**b**, **d**, **f**) are shown. The *arrowhead* in **d** points toward the abnormally shaped dorsal root entry zones in Sox10$^{Dom/Dom}$ mutants; *arrows* in **a** and **e** point towards B-FABP-positive Schwann cell precursors that line spinal nerves in control and ErbB3$^{-/-}$ mice (Picture reproduced by permission of Cold Spring Harbor Laboratory Press.)

determined whether both Sox10 and the Delta/Notch pathway interact in the control of glial cell differentiation.

The genes encoding for P$_0$ and Connexin 32 have been shown to be direct transcriptional targets of Sox10. Both genes are associated with the late differentiation and the formation of myelin in Schwann cells (Abrams et al. 2000; Peirano et al. 2000; Bondurand et al. 2001; Lobsiger et al. 2002; Suter and Scherer 2003). This indicates that Sox10 exerts sequential functions during different phases of peripheral glial development. Indeed, mutations of the SOX10 gene in humans have been found to be associated with myelination defects in peripheral nerves, similar to Charcot-Marie-Tooth syndrome type I, a disease state typically associated with Schwann cell defects (Kuhlbrodt et al. 1998b; Pingault et al. 1998; Bondurand et al. 1999; Inoue et al. 1999; Pingault et al. 2000; Touraine et al. 2000; Bondurand et al. 2001; Pingault et al. 2001; Berger et al. 2002; Maier et al. 2002; Suter and Scherer 2003).

The transcription factor Sox10 and the Neuregulin-1/ErbB2/ErbB3 pathway control Schwann cell development through overlapping as well as separate molecular mechanisms. The mutation of these genes in mice results in an identical phenotype, however, which is characterized by the complete ablation of Schwann cells from the peripheral nervous system. Neuregulin-1-signaling mutants develop a severe degeneration of motor neurons which has been interpreted as secondary to the loss of Schwann cells that may provide accompanying motor axons with survival signals (for detailed discussion see Sect. 2.2.1.2; Riethmacher et al. 1997; Woldeyesus et al. 1999; Wolpowitz et al. 2000). Unlike Sox10, which is expressed only by glial cells in the developing peripheral nervous system, components of the Neuregulin-1/ErbB2/ErbB3 pathway are expressed at the muscle targets as well, and muscle innervation is impaired in Neuregulin-1-signaling mutants (Yang et al. 1998; Morris et al. 1999; Woldeyesus et al. 1999; Wolpowitz et al. 2000). Owing to this, it was argued that genetic ablation of Neuregulin-1, or its specific receptors in the peripheral nervous system, might also affect neuronal survival via altering expression of target-derived neurotrophic factors (Bibel and Barde 2000). Mice with mutation of the Sox10 gene, however, develop degeneration of motor neurons indistinguishable in its time-course and distribution along the neuroaxis from the neuropathies observed in Neuregulin-1-signaling mutants (Fig. 9; Riethmacher et al. 1997; Woldeyesus et al. 1999; Britsch et al. 2001). This unambiguously demonstrated that the lack of Schwann cells and Schwann-cell-dependent signals acting on accompanying axons is responsible for neuronal degeneration in mice with mutations of ErbB2, ErbB3, or Neuregulin-1 (Britsch et al. 2001). Presumably, this survival signal corresponds to a specific function of a particular isoform of Neuregulin-1, the type III isoform. Unlike type I or II, type III is critical for Schwann cell development and the maintenance of adjacent axons (Meyer and Birchmeier 1995; Kramer et al. 1996; Meyer et al. 1997; Wolpowitz et al. 2000). It is the only isoform expressed on axon membranes, and this isoform has been demonstrated in vitro to allow bi-directional signaling (Bermingham-McDonogh et al. 1997; Yang et al. 1998; Bao et al. 2003).

One of the most interesting questions in the field is the direct in vivo assessment of the molecular nature of these Schwann-cell-dependent neuronal survival signals.

## 2.4
## NRG-1/ErbB Signals and Disease

### 2.4.1
### ErbB Receptors in Cancer and Heart Disease

ErbB2 was originally identified because of its oncogenic potential (Hynes and Stern 1994; Olayioye et al. 2000). It was Robert Weinberg's lab that first observed the neu-oncogene to be activated in neuro- and glioblastomas derived from rats treated with the mutagen ethylnitrosourea (EtNU); they showed the neu-oncogene to encode an EGFR-related transmembrane tyrosine kinase receptor (Bargmann et al. 1986). Mutagenesis of rats with ethylnitrosourea was also observed to induce Schwannomas of the trigeminal nerve with high frequency. In all Schwannomas, an identical point mutation at position 2012 of the ErbB2 gene occurs. This mutation leads to the exchange of a single amino acid within the transmembrane domain of ErbB2 (Nikitin et al. 1991). Introduction of the oncogenic variant of ErbB2 into NIH3T3 cells has been shown to induce their malignant transformation (Bargmann et al. 1986). Moreover, overexpression of a nonmutated ErbB2 proto-oncogene in fibroblasts suffices to transform these cells (Di Fiore et al. 1987). Overexpression of ErbB2 as a consequence of gene amplification was first detected in human mammary carcinomas (King et al. 1985). Since then it has been observed in many different human malignancies (Hynes and Stern 1994; Holbro et al. 2003; Holbro and Hynes 2004). Overexpression of ErbB2 correlates with relapse and survival of patients with breast or ovarian cancer (Slamon et al. 1987; Slamon et al. 1989). Transgenic expression of the activated, oncogenic variant of ErbB2, and the overexpression of unactivated ErbB2 in mice under the transcriptional control of the mouse mammary tumor virus (MMTV) promoter/enhancer results in the induction of mammary tumors that can metastasize, providing direct evidence in vivo for the critical role of ErbB2 in tumor induction (Muller et al. 1988; Bouchard et al. 1989; Guy et al. 1992).

Overexpression of ErbB2 is thought to result in ligand-independent activation of its kinase domain through spontaneous dimer formation. Cooperation of ErbB receptors, however, has been described in oncogenic transformation, both in vitro and in primary human tumors, and this mechanism may contribute to tumor development as well, since coexpression of ErbB2 and ErbB1 as well as of ErbB2 and ErbB3 can synergize in transformation and tumorigenic growth in vitro (Kokai et al. 1989; Alimandi et al. 1995; Wallasch et al. 1995). Furthermore, transgenic mice overexpressing neu have been shown to overexpress endogenous ErbB1, and the loss of ErbB2 function inhibits the growth of tumor cells with an autocrine activation of ErbB1 (Jannot et al. 1996; DiGiovanna et al. 1998). This is in line with a recent clinical study reporting the poorest prognosis in breast cancer patients coexpressing ErbB2 and ErbB1 (DiGiovanna et al. 2005). Coexpression of ErbB2 and ErbB4 occurs in >50% of childhood medulloblastomas and a significant proportion of these tumors express the corresponding ligand Neuregulin-1 (Gilbertson et al. 1997; Gilbertson et al. 1998).

Due to its oncogenic potential and its involvement in many types of human cancer, the ErbB2 receptor has received great attention as a diagnostic parameter in clinical medicine and as a target for therapeutic intervention (Hynes and Lane 2005). For example, identification of ErbB2 amplification by fluorescent in situ hybridization (FISH) has been approved by the FDA to identify patients at high risk for relapse and disease-associated death with invasive mammary carcinoma (Press et al. 1997; Ross and Fletcher 1998). Other clinical studies have been able to correlate the ErbB2 receptor state with the therapeutic response in breast cancer (Borg et al. 1994; Muss et al. 1994).

Several strategies have been pursued to target therapeutically ErbB2. The most promising and advanced strategies include small chemical inhibitors that can interfere with tyrosine kinase activity of ErbB2, and monoclonal antibodies directed against ErbB2 that inhibit its function (Holbro and Hynes 2004; Hynes and Lane 2005). A monoclonal antibody, 4D5, which targets the extracellular domain of ErbB2, has been first demonstrated to inhibit effectively the growth of ErbB2-overexpressing tumor cells in vitro (Hudziak et al. 1989; Lewis et al. 1993; Lewis et al. 1996). A fully humanized version of this antibody (Trastuzumab, Herceptin, Genentech/Roche, Basel) was clinically validated and is now a standard therapeutic tool, both alone or in combination with chemotherapeutic agents in patients with metastatic breast cancer overexpressing ErbB2 (Baselga et al. 1996; Pegram et al. 1998; Cobleigh et al. 1999). Herceptin inhibits receptor activation and downstream signaling pathways and has been shown to promote receptor internalization. This results in an antiproliferative effect of Herceptin on tumor cells, the downregulation of positive cell cycle regulators, and an increase of inhibitors, such as the cyclin-dependent kinase inhibitor p27[Kip1] (Sliwkowski et al. 1999). Furthermore, Herceptin has been shown to recruit immune effector cells to ErbB2-overexpressing tumors, which may contribute to its mechanism of action (Clynes et al. 2000).

Another anti-ErbB2 mononclonal antibody, 2C4 (Pertuzumab, Omnitarg, Genentech/Roche), is currently evaluated in a Phase II trial for treatment of ovarian cancer. Unlike Herceptin, which does not bind to a region of ErbB2 involved in receptor heterodimerization (Cho et al. 2003), Omnitarg binds to the extracellular domain II of ErbB2 (Agus et al. 2002; Franklin et al. 2004). This domain is critical for receptor dimerization (Burgess et al. 2003). As a consequence, Omnitarg interferes with heterodimer formation and downstream signaling, while Herceptin is unable to block heterodimerization of ErbB2 (Agus et al. 2002; Franklin et al. 2004). The nonoverlapping mechanisms of action of both antibodies result in differential anti-tumor activity, with Omnitarg but not Herceptin being still active in tumors that express low levels of ErbB2 (Agus et al. 2002). Omnitarg probably inhibits auto- or paracrine signaling through ErbB2 heterodimers in these tumors. Hence, Pertuzumab represents a promising novel therapeutic agent, which may help in the future to complement the therapeutic spectrum of Herceptin, especially in tumors where cooperation of ErbB2 with additional ErbBs occurs (Baselga 2002; Badache and Hynes 2004).

Herceptin increases the survival of patients suffering from breast cancer, when combined with first-line conventional chemotherapy. However, when coadministered with anthracyclines or given to patients that had previously received chemotherapy with these drugs, Herceptin treatment is associated with increased risk for cardiac side effects, including cardiac dysfunction (Slamon et al. 2001; Seidman et al. 2002). These clinical observations provide a remarkable link to mouse genetics: (1) targeted deletion of components of the Neuregulin-1/ErbB signaling pathway results in embryonic death due to defective heart development with the loss of trabeculation and the pumping failure of the embryonic heart (Gassmann et al. 1995; Lee et al. 1995; Meyer and Birchmeier 1995; Kramer et al. 1996; Britsch et al. 1998; Liu et al. 1998); (2) heart-specific ablation of ErbB2 in adult mice leads to clinical symptoms resembling dilatated cardiomyopathy (DCMDCM); and (3) furthermore, cardiomyocytes derived from ErbB2 mutant mice display increased sensitivity to anthracycline-induced cytotoxicity (Crone et al. 2002; Ozcelik et al. 2002; Garratt et al. 2003; Negro et al. 2004). Thus, animals with heart-specific ablation of ErbB2 provide valuable disease models that will help to assess novel therapeutic agents interfering with ErbB2 function. In the end, such animal models will also allow better understanding of the molecular mechanisms underlying development of dilated cardiomyopathy (Chien and Olson 2002; Ozcelik et al. 2002; Negro et al. 2004).

## 2.4.2
### Neuregulin-1 and Susceptibility to Schizophrenia

Schizophrenia is a severe psychiatric disorder with a lifetime risk of 0.5–1%. The disease is characterized by psychotic symptoms, reduced interest and motivation, altered emotional reactivity, and disorganized behavior. Affected individuals often show subtle cognitive and social deficits preceding the first manifestation of disease, which can occur in early childhood. Typically, schizophrenia is a relapsing disorder with episodes of only partial remission and produces life-long disability (Owen et al. 2005). Early onset of initial symptoms and the lack of obvious signs of neurodegeneration in affected individuals have lead to a revised view of the pathology of schizophrenia, which is now more often considered to be a neurodevelopmental disorder (Corfas et al. 2004). Although family and twin studies have unambiguously demonstrated an increased risk of illness for relatives of patients suffering from schizophrenia, with heritability rates as high as approx. 80%, it is clear that environmental factors contribute significantly to the pathogenesis of the disease. Various susceptibility loci on different chromosomes have been identified, suggesting more than one gene to be involved in the susceptibility to the disorder. A genome-wide linkage analysis in the Icelandic population first identified the Neuregulin-1 gene to be associated with a susceptibility locus for schizophrenia (Stefansson et al. 2002). Several follow-up studies from different populations as well as a meta-analysis of the existing association studies confirmed this observation (Lohmueller et al. 2003; Yang et al. 2003; Corvin et al. 2004; Hall et al. 2004; Li et al. 2004; Tang et al. 2004; Zhao et al. 2004). However, in some studies no association between Neuregulin-1 and schizophrenia was found (Hong et al. 2004; Iwata et al. 2004; Thiselton et al. 2004). No specific susceptibility variants or mutations of the Neuregulin-1 gene have been identified in the susceptibility loci (Stefansson et al. 2002). The Neuregulin-1 gene is known to employ different promoters and extensive alternative splicing, thereby giving rise to many different isoforms. Since the Icelandic haplotype localizes to the 5' end of the Neuregulin-1 gene, altered gene expression or mRNA splicing have been suggested to be involved in disease susceptibility (Owen et al. 2005). In support of this, altered ratios of three mRNA isoforms of Neuregulin-1 have been observed in the prefrontal cortex of schizophrenic patients (Hashimoto et al. 2004). The genomic region of the human Neuregulin-1 gene, as well as flanking regions do not harbor additional known genes. Therefore, it is unlikely that genes in the close neighborhood of Neuregulin-1 are linked to the disease susceptibility. Nonetheless, there is some recent evidence that the first intron of the human Neuregulin-1 gene contains an expressed sequence of unknown function (Corvin et al. 2004). Mice lacking one copy of the Neuregulin-1 gene have been shown to be hyperactive and to have deficits in prepulse inhibition (Gerlai et al. 2000; Stefansson et al. 2002). Both behavioral abnormalities are related to symptoms found in schizophrenic patients. Interestingly, hyperactivity improves when heterozygous Neuregulin-1 mutant mice are treated with antipsychotic drugs (Stefansson et al. 2002). Further indication for the Neuregulin-1/ErbB pathway being involved in schizophrenia comes from the observation that ErbB3 expression in the prefrontal cortex of schizophrenics is significantly reduced. However, since many oligodendrocyte-associated genes have been described to be reduced in affected patients, reduction of ErbB3 might not be causative but reflect a more general oligodendrocyte dysfunction (Hakak et al. 2001; Tkachev et al. 2003).

At present, it is absolutely unclear by which mechanisms altered Neuregulin-1 function might contribute to schizophrenia. However, this signaling pathway has been implicated in processes such as neuronal migration and differentiation, synapse formation, neuronal connectivity, and myelination—processes that have been linked to schizophrenia as well. The availability of mouse models with brain-specific mutations of the Neuregulin-1-signaling pathway together with a broadened repertoire of behavioral, structural, and imaging analyses will allow a systematic assessment of the functions of this gene in the context of mental disease (Corfas et al. 2004; Stefansson et al. 2004).

# 3
# Summary

Neuregulins (NRGs) comprise a large family of EGF-like signaling molecules involved in cell–cell communication during development and disease. The neuregulin family of ligands has four members: NRG1, NRG2, NRG3, and NRG4. Relatively little is known about the biological functions of the NRG2, 3, and 4 proteins. In contrast, the NRG1 proteins have been demonstrated to play important roles during the development of the nervous system, heart, and mammary glands. For example, NRG1 has essential functions in the development of neural crest cells and some of their major derivatives, like Schwann cells and sympathetic neurons. NRG1 controls the trabeculation of the myocardial musculature and the ductal differentiation of the mammary epithelium. Moreover, there is emerging evidence for the involvement of NRG signals in the development and function of several other organ systems, and in human disease, including breast cancer and schizophrenia. Many different isoforms of the Neuregulin-1 gene are synthesized. Such isoforms differ in their tissue-specific expression patterns and their biological activities, thereby contributing to the great diversity of the in vivo functions of NRG1.

Neuregulins transmit their signals to target cells by interacting with transmembrane tyrosine kinase receptors of the ErbB family. This family includes four members, the epidermal growth factor receptor (EGF-R, ErbB1, ErbB2, ErbB3, and ErbB4). Receptor-ligand interaction induces the heterodimerization of receptor monomers, which in turn results in the activation of intracellular signaling cascades and the induction of cellular responses including proliferation, migration, differentiation, and survival or apoptosis. In vivo, functional NRG1 receptors are heterodimers composed of ErbB2 with either an ErbB3, or ErbB4 molecule. The tissue-specific distribution of the different receptor types further contributes to the diversity and specificity of the biological functions of this signaling pathway.

It is a typical feature of the Neuregulin-1/ErbB signaling pathway to control sequential steps during the development of a particular organ system. For example, this pathway functions in early precursor proliferation, maturation, as well as in the myelination of Schwann cells. The systematic analysis of genetic models that have been established by the help of conventional as well as conditional gene targeting strategies in mice was instrumental for the uncovering of the multitude of biological functions of this signaling system. In this review the basic biology of the Neuregulin-1/ErbB system and how it relates to the in vivo functions were discussed with special emphasis to transgenic techniques in mice.

# References

Abrams CK, Oh S, Ri Y, Bargiello TA (2000) Mutations in connexin 32: the molecular and biophysical bases for the X-linked form of Charcot-Marie-Tooth disease. Brain Res Brain Res Rev 32:203–14.

Adlkofer K, Lai C (2000) Role of neuregulins in glial cell development. Glia 29:104–11.

Agus DB, Akita RW, Fox WD, Lewis GD, Higgins B, Pisacane PI, Lofgren JA, Tindell C, Evans DP, Maiese K, Scher HI, Sliwkowski MX (2002) Targeting ligand-activated ErbB2 signaling inhibits breast and prostate tumor growth. Cancer Cell 2:127–37.

Akiyama H, Chaboissier MC, Martin JF, Schedl A, de Crombrugghe B (2002) The transcription factor Sox9 has essential roles in successive steps of the chondrocyte differentiation pathway and is required for expression of Sox5 and Sox6. Genes Dev 16:2813–28.

Alimandi M, Romano A, Curia MC, Muraro R, Fedi P, Aaronson SA, Di Fiore PP, Kraus MH (1995) Cooperative signaling of ErbB3 and ErbB2 in neoplastic transformation and human mammary carcinomas. Oncogene 10:1813–21.

Altiok N, Bessereau JL, Changeux JP (1995) ErbB3 and ErbB2/neu mediate the effect of heregulin on acetylcholine receptor gene expression in muscle: differential expression at the endplate. Embo J 14:4258–66.

Alvarez-Buylla A, Seri B, Doetsch F (2002) Identification of neural stem cells in the adult vertebrate brain. Brain Res Bull 57:751–8.

Anderson DJ, Groves A, Lo L, Ma Q, Rao M, Shah NM, Sommer L (1997) Cell lineage determination and the control of neuronal identity in the neural crest. Cold Spring Harb Symp Quant Biol 62:493–504.

Anderson KV, Ingham PW (2003) The transformation of the model organism: a decade of developmental genetics. Nat Genet 33 Suppl:285–93.

Andrechek ER, Hardy WR, Girgis-Gabardo AA, Perry RL, Butler R, Graham FL, Kahn RC, Rudnicki MA, Muller WJ (2002) ErbB2 is required for muscle spindle and myoblast cell survival. Mol Cell Biol 22:4714–22.

Anton ES, Ghashghaei HT, Weber JL, McCann C, Fischer TM, Cheung ID, Gassmann M, Messing A, Klein R, Schwab MH, Lloyd KC, Lai C (2004) Receptor tyrosine kinase ErbB4 modulates neuroblast migration and placement in the adult forebrain. Nat Neurosci 7:1319–28.

Arber S, Ladle DR, Lin JH, Frank E, Jessell TM (2000) ETS gene Er81 controls the formation of functional connections between group Ia sensory afferents and motor neurons. Cell 101:485–98.

Aroian RV, Koga M, Mendel JE, Ohshima Y, Sternberg PW (1990) The let-23 gene necessary for Caenorhabditis elegans vulval induction encodes a tyrosine kinase of the EGF receptor subfamily. Nature 348:693–9.

Aroian, and RV Sternberg PW (1991) Multiple functions of let-23, a Caenorhabditis elegans receptor tyrosine kinase gene required for vulval induction. Genetics 128:251–67.

Artavanis-Tsakonas S, Rand MD, Lake RJ (1999) Notch signaling: cell fate control and signal integration in development. Science 284:770–6.

Asakura M, Kitakaze M, Takashima S, Liao Y, Ishikura F, Yoshinaka T, Ohmoto H, Node K, Yoshino K, Ishiguro H, Asanuma H, Sanada S, Matsumura Y, Takeda H, Beppu S, Tada M, Hori M, Higashiyama S (2002) Cardiac hypertrophy is inhibited by antagonism of ADAM12 processing of HB-EGF: metalloproteinase inhibitors as a new therapy. Nat Med 8:35–40.

Badache A, Hynes NE (2004) A new therapeutic antibody masks ErbB2 to its partners. Cancer Cell 5:299–301.

Baker NE (2000) Notch signaling in the nervous system. Pieces still missing from the puzzle. Bioessays 22:264–73.

Baliga RR, Pimental DR, Zhao YY, Simmons WW, Marchionni MA, Sawyer DB, Kelly RA (1999) NRG-1-induced cardiomyocyte hypertrophy. Role of PI-3-kinase, p70(S6 K), and MEK-MAPK-RSK. Am J Physiol 277:H2026–37.

Bao J, Wolpowitz D, Role LW, Talmage DA (2003) Back signaling by the Nrg-1 intracellular domain. J Cell Biol 161:1133–41.

Barembaum M, Bronner-Fraser M (2005) Early steps in neural crest specification. Semin Cell Dev Biol 16:642–6.

Bargmann CI, Hung MC, Weinberg RA (1986) The neu oncogene encodes an epidermal growth factor receptor-related protein. Nature 319:226–30.

Barres BA, Raff MC (1999) Axonal control of oligodendrocyte development. J Cell Biol 147:1123–8.

Baselga J (2002) A new anti-ErbB2 strategy in the treatment of cancer: prevention of ligand-dependent ErbB2 receptor heterodimerization. Cancer Cell 2:93–5.

Baselga J, Tripathy D, Mendelsohn J, Baughman S, Benz CC, Dantis L, Sklarin NT, Seidman AD, Hudis CA, Moore J, Rosen PP, Twaddell T, Henderson IC, Norton L (1996) Phase II study of weekly intravenous recombinant humanized anti- p185HER2 monoclonal antibody in patients with HER2/neu-overexpressing metastatic breast cancer. J Clin Oncol 14:737–44.

Berger P, Young P, Suter U (2002) Molecular cell biology of Charcot-Marie-Tooth disease. Neurogenetics 4:1–15.

Bermingham-McDonogh O, Xu YT, Marchionni MA, Scherer SS (1997) Neuregulin expression in PNS neurons: isoforms and regulation by target interactions. Mol Cell Neurosci 10:184–95.

Bibel M, Barde YA (2000) Neurotrophins: key regulators of cell fate and cell shape in the vertebrate nervous system. Genes Dev 14:2919–37.

Biscardi JS, Maa MC, Tice DA, Cox ME, Leu TH, Parsons SJ (1999) c-Src-mediated phosphorylation of the epidermal growth factor receptor on Tyr845 and Tyr1101 is associated with modulation of receptor function. J Biol Chem 274:8335–43.

Bondurand N, Girard M, Pingault V, Lemort N, Dubourg O, Goossens M (2001) Human Connexin 32, a gap junction protein altered in the X-linked form of Charcot-Marie-Tooth disease, is directly regulated by the transcription factor SOX10. Hum Mol Genet 10:2783–95.

Bondurand N, Kuhlbrodt K, Pingault V, Enderich J, Sajus M, Tommerup N, Warburg M, Hennekam RC, Read AP, Wegner M, Goossens M (1999) A molecular analysis of the Yemenite deaf-blind hypopigmentation syndrome: SOX10 dysfunction causes different neurocristopathies. Hum Mol Genet 8:1785–9.

Borg A, Baldetorp B, Ferno M, Killander D, Olsson H, Ryden S, Sigurdsson H (1994) ERBB2 amplification is associated with tamoxifen resistance in steroid-receptor positive breast cancer. Cancer Lett 81:137–44.

Bouchard L, Lamarre L, Tremblay PJ, Jolicoeur P (1989) Stochastic appearance of mammary tumors in transgenic mice carrying the MMTV/c-neu oncogene. Cell 57:931–6.

Britsch S (2006) Transgenic and knockout animals. In: Encyclopedic Reference of Genomics and Proteomics in Molecular Medicine (ed. Ganten D, Ruckpaul K). Springer Verlag, Heidelberg, New York.

Britsch S, Goerich DE, Riethmacher D, Peirano RI, Rossner M, Nave KA, Birchmeier C, Wegner M (2001) The transcription factor Sox10 is a key regulator of peripheral glial development. Genes Dev 15:66–78.

Britsch S, Li L, Kirchhoff S, Theuring F, Brinkmann V, Birchmeier C, Riethmacher D (1998) The ErbB2 and ErbB3 receptors and their ligand, neuregulin-1, are essential for development of the sympathetic nervous system. Genes Dev 12:1825–36.

Britsch S, Strehle M, Birchmeier C (2003) Tiermodelle in der Biomedizinischen Forschung. In: Handbuch der Molekularen Medizin, Bd. 1, Molekular und Zellbiologische Grundlagen (ed. Ganten D, Ruckpaul K). Springer Verlag, Heidelberg, New York.

Britto JM, Lukehurst S, Weller R, Fraser C, Qiu Y, Hertzog P, Busfield SJ (2004) Generation and characterization of neuregulin-2-deficient mice. Mol Cell Biol 24:8221–6.

Brockes JP, Lemke GE, Balzer DR, Jr. (1980) Purification and preliminary characterization of a glial growth factor from the bovine pituitary. J Biol Chem 255:8374–7.

Bunge RP (1993) Expanding roles for the Schwann cell: ensheathment, myelination, trophism and regeneration. Curr Opin Neurobiol 3:805–9.

Buonanno A, Fischbach GD (2001) Neuregulin and ErbB receptor signaling pathways in the nervous system. Curr Opin Neurobiol 11:287–96.

Burden S, Yarden Y (1997) Neuregulins and their receptors: a versatile signaling module in organogenesis and oncogenesis. Neuron 18:847–55.

Burgess AW, Cho HS, Eigenbrot C, Ferguson KM, Garrett TP, Leahy DJ, Lemmon MA, Sliwkowski MX, Ward CW, Yokoyama S (2003) An open-and-shut case? Recent insights into the activation of EGF/ErbB receptors. Mol Cell 12:541–52.

Busfield SJ, Michnick DA, Chickering TW, Revett TL, Ma J, Woolf EA, Comrack CA, Dussault BJ, Woolf J, Goodearl AD, Gearing DP (1997) Characterization of a neuregulin-related gene, Don-1, that is highly expressed in restricted regions of the cerebellum and hippocampus. Mol Cell Biol 17:4007–14.

Calaora V, Rogister B, Bismuth K, Murray K, Brandt H, Leprince P, Marchionni M, Dubois-Dalcq M (2001) Neuregulin signaling regulates neural precursor growth and the generation of oligodendrocytes in vitro. J Neurosci 21:4740–51.

Camenisch TD, Schroeder JA, Bradley J, Klewer SE, McDonald JA (2002) Heart-valve mesenchyme formation is dependent on hyaluronan-augmented activation of ErbB2-ErbB3 receptors. Nat Med 8:850–5.

Cannella B, Pitt D, Marchionni M, Raine CS (1999) Neuregulin and erbB receptor expression in normal and diseased human white matter. J Neuroimmunol 100:233–42.

Canoll PD, Musacchio JM, Hardy R, Reynolds R, Marchionni MA, Salzer JL (1996) GGF/neuregulin is a neuronal signal that promotes the proliferation and survival and inhibits the differentiation of oligodendrocyte progenitors. Neuron 17:229–43.

Carpenter G (2000) EGF receptor transactivation mediated by the proteolytic production of EGF-like agonists. Sci STKE 2000:PE1.

Carraway KL, 3rd, Weber JL, Unger MJ, Ledesma J, Yu N, Gassmann M, Lai C (1997) Neuregulin-2, a new ligand of ErbB3/ErbB4-receptor tyrosine kinases. Nature 387:512–6.

Carraway KL, Ramsauer VP, Haq B, Carothers Carraway CA (2003) Cell signaling through membrane mucins. Bioessays 25:66–71.

Carraway KR, Cantley LC (1994) A neu acquaintance for erbB3 and erbB4: a role for receptor heterodimerization in growth signaling. Cell 78:5–8.

Carraway KR, Sliwkowski MX, Akita R, Platko JV, Guy PM, Nuijens A, Diamonti AJ, Vandlen RL, Cantley LC, Cerione RA (1994) The erbB3 gene product is a receptor for heregulin. J Biol Chem 269:14303–6.

Chang H, Riese DJ, 2nd, Gilbert W, Stern DF, McMahan UJ (1997) Ligands for ErbB-family receptors encoded by a neuregulin-like gene. Nature 387:509–12.

Chen MS, Bermingham-McDonogh O, Danehy FT, Jr., Nolan C, Scherer SS, Lucas J, Gwynne D, Marchionni MA (1994) Expression of multiple neuregulin transcripts in postnatal rat brains. J Comp Neurol 349:389–400.

Chen S, Rio C, Ji RR, Dikkes P, Coggeshall RE, Woolf CJ, Corfas G (2003) Disruption of ErbB receptor signaling in adult non-myelinating Schwann cells causes progressive sensory loss. Nat Neurosci. 6:1186–93

Cheung M, Briscoe J (2003) Neural crest development is regulated by the transcription factor Sox9. Development 130:5681–93.

Cheung M, Chaboissier MC, Mynett A, Hirst E, Schedl A, Briscoe J (2005) The transcriptional control of trunk neural crest induction, survival, and delamination. Dev Cell 8:179–92.

Chien KR, Olson EN (2002) Converging pathways and principles in heart development and disease: CV@CSH. Cell 110:153–62.

Cho HS, Mason K, Ramyar KX, Stanley AM, Gabelli SB, Denney DW, Jr., and Leahy DJ (2003) Structure of the extracellular region of HER2 alone and in complex with the Herceptin Fab. Nature 421:756–60.

Citri A, Skaria KB, Yarden Y (2003) The deaf and the dumb: the biology of ErbB-2 and ErbB-3. Exp Cell Res 284:54–65.

Civenni G, Holbro T, Hynes NE (2003) Wnt1 and Wnt5a induce cyclin D1 expression through ErbB1 transactivation in HC11 mammary epithelial cells. EMBO Rep 4:166–71.

Clynes RA, Towers TL, Presta LG, Ravetch JV (2000) Inhibitory Fc receptors modulate in vivo cytotoxicity against tumor targets. Nat Med 6:443–6.

Cobleigh MA, Vogel CL, Tripathy D, Robert NJ, Scholl S, Fehrenbacher L, Wolter JM, Paton V, Shak S, Lieberman G, Slamon DJ (1999) Multinational study of the efficacy and safety of humanized anti-HER2 monoclonal antibody in women who have HER2-overexpressing metastatic breast cancer that has progressed after chemotherapy for metastatic disease. J Clin Oncol 17:2639–48.

Corfas G, Rosen KM, Aratake H, Krauss R, Fischbach GD (1995) Differential expression of ARIA isoforms in the rat brain. Neuron 14:103–15.

Corfas G, Roy K, Buxbaum JD (2004) Neuregulin 1-erbB signaling and the molecular/cellular basis of schizophrenia. Nat Neurosci 7:575–80.

Corvin AP, Morris DW, McGhee K, Schwaiger S, Scully P, Quinn J, Meagher D, Clair DS, Waddington JL, Gill M (2004) Confirmation and refinement of an 'at-risk' haplotype for schizophrenia suggests the EST cluster, Hs.97362, as a potential susceptibility gene at the Neuregulin-1 locus. Mol Psychiatry 9:208–13.

Crone SA, Zhao YY, Fan L, Gu Y, Minamisawa S, Liu Y, Peterson KL, Chen J, Kahn R, Condorelli G, Ross J, Jr., Chien KR, Lee KF (2002) ErbB2 is essential in the prevention of dilated cardiomyopathy. Nat Med 8:459–65.

Daub H, Weiss FU, Wallasch C, Ullrich A (1996) Role of transactivation of the EGF receptor in signalling by G-protein-coupled receptors. Nature 379:557–60.

del Barrio MG, Nieto MA (2002) Overexpression of Snail family members highlights their ability to promote chick neural crest formation. Development 129:1583–93.

Di Fiore PP, Pierce JH, Kraus MH, Segatto O, King CR, Aaronson SA (1987) erbB-2 is a potent oncogene when overexpressed in NIH/3T3 cells. Science 237:178–82.

DiGiovanna MP, Lerman MA, Coffey RJ, Muller WJ, Cardiff RD, Stern DF (1998) Active signaling by Neu in transgenic mice. Oncogene 17:1877–84.

DiGiovanna MP, Stern DF, Edgerton SM, Whalen SG, Moore D, 2nd, Thor AD (2005) Relationship of epidermal growth factor receptor expression to ErbB-2 signaling activity and prognosis in breast cancer patients. J Clin Oncol 23:1152–60.

Doetsch F, Garcia-Verdugo JM, Alvarez-Buylla A (1997) Cellular composition and three-dimensional organization of the subventricular germinal zone in the adult mammalian brain. J Neurosci 17:5046–61.

Dong Z, Brennan A, Liu N, Yarden Y, Lefkowitz G, Mirsky R, Jessen KR (1995) Neu differentiation factor is a neuron-glia signal and regulates survival, proliferation, and maturation of rat Schwann cell precursors. Neuron 15:585–96.

Donovan MJ, Lin MI, Wiegn P, Ringstedt T, Kraemer R, Hahn R, Wang S, Ibanez CF, Rafii S, Hempstead BL (2000) Brain derived neurotrophic factor is an endothelial cell survival factor required for intramyocardial vessel stabilization. Development 127:4531–40.

Dottori M, Gross MK, Labosky P, Goulding M (2001) The winged-helix transcription factor Foxd3 suppresses interneuron differentiation and promotes neural crest cell fate. Development 128:4127–38.

Dowsing BJ, Morrison WA, Nicola NA, Starkey GP, Bucci T, Kilpatrick TJ (1999) Leukemia inhibitory factor is an autocrine survival factor for Schwann cells. J Neurochem 73:96–104.

Durbec PL, Larsson-Blomberg LB, Schuchardt A, Costantini F, Pachnis V (1996) Common origin and developmental dependence on c-ret of subsets of enteric and sympathetic neuroblasts. Development 122:349–58.

Erickson SL, O'Shea KS, Ghaboosi N, Loverro L, Frantz G, Bauer M, Lu LH, Moore MW (1997) ErbB3 is required for normal cerebellar and cardiac development: a comparison with ErbB2-and heregulin-deficient mice. Development 124:4999–5011.

Ernfors P, Lee KF, Kucera J, Jaenisch R (1994) Lack of neurotrophin-3 leads to deficiencies in the peripheral nervous system and loss of limb proprioceptive afferents. Cell 77:503–12.

Escher P, Lacazette E, Courtet M, Blindenbacher A, Landmann L, Bezakova G, Lloyd KC, Mueller U, Brenner HR (2005) Synapses form in skeletal muscles lacking neuregulin receptors. Science 308:1920–3.

Falls DL (2003) Neuregulins: functions, forms, and signaling strategies. Exp Cell Res 284:14–30.

Falls DL, Rosen KM, Corfas G, Lane WS, Fischbach GD (1993) ARIA, a protein that stimulates acetylcholine receptor synthesis, is a member of the neu ligand family. Cell 72:801–15.

Fernandez PA, Tang DG, Cheng L, Prochiantz A, Mudge AW, Raff MC (2000) Evidence that axon-derived neuregulin promotes oligodendrocyte survival in the developing rat optic nerve. Neuron 28:81–90.

Fischbach GD, Rosen KM (1997) ARIA: a neuromuscular junction neuregulin. Annu Rev Neurosci 20:429–58.

Flames N, Long JE, Garratt AN, Fischer TM, Gassmann M, Birchmeier C, Lai C, Rubenstein JL, Marin O (2004) Short- and long-range attraction of cortical GABAergic interneurons by neuregulin-1. Neuron 44:251–61.

Flames N, Marin O (2005) Developmental mechanisms underlying the generation of cortical interneuron diversity. Neuron 46:377–81.

Francis N, Farinas I, Brennan C, Rivas-Plata K, Backus C, Reichardt L, Landis S (1999) NT-3, like NGF, is required for survival of sympathetic neurons, but not their precursors. Dev Biol 210:411–27.

Franklin MC, Carey KD, Vajdos FF, Leahy DJ, de Vos AM, Sliwkowski MX (2004) Insights into ErbB signaling from the structure of the ErbB2-pertuzumab complex. Cancer Cell 5:317–28.

Gage FH (2002) Neurogenesis in the adult brain. J Neurosci 22:612–3.

Gammill LS, Bronner-Fraser M (2002) Genomic analysis of neural crest induction. Development 129:5731–41.

Gammill LS, Gonzalez C, Gu C, Bronner-Fraser M (2005) Guidance of trunk neural crest migration requires neuropilin 2/semaphorin 3F signaling. Development. 133:99–106

Garcia-Castro MI, Marcelle C, Bronner-Fraser M (2002) Ectodermal Wnt function as a neural crest inducer. Science 297:848–51.

Garratt AN, Britsch S, Birchmeier C (2000a) Neuregulin, a factor with many functions in the life of a Schwann cell. Bioessays 22:987–96.

Garratt AN, Ozcelik C, Birchmeier C (2003) ErbB2 pathways in heart and neural diseases. Trends Cardiovasc Med 13:80–6.

Garratt AN, Voiculescu O, Topilko P, Charnay P, Birchmeier C (2000b) A dual role of erbB2 in myelination and in expansion of the Schwann cell precursor pool. J Cell Biol 148:1035–46.

Garrett TP, McKern NM, Lou M, Elleman TC, Adams TE, Lovrecz GO, Kofler M, Jorissen RN, Nice EC, Burgess AW, Ward CW (2003) The crystal structure of a truncated ErbB2 ectodomain reveals an active conformation, poised to interact with other ErbB receptors. Mol Cell 11:495–505.

Garrett TP, McKern NM, Lou M, Elleman TC, Adams TE, Lovrecz GO, Zhu HJ, Walker F, Frenkel MJ, Hoyne PA, Jorissen RN, Nice EC, Burgess AW, Ward CW (2002) Crystal structure of a truncated epidermal growth factor receptor extracellular domain bound to transforming growth factor alpha. Cell 110:763–73.

Gassmann M, Casagranda F, Orioli D, Simon H, Lai C, Klein R, Lemke G (1995) Aberrant neural and cardiac development in mice lacking the erbb4 neuregulin receptor. Nature 378:390–394.

Gerlai R, Pisacane P, Erickson S (2000) Heregulin, but not ErbB2 or ErbB3, heterozygous mutant mice exhibit hyperactivity in multiple behavioral tasks. Behav Brain Res 109:219–27.

Gilbertson RJ, Clifford SC, MacMeekin W, Meekin W, Wright C, Perry RH, Kelly P, Pearson AD, Lunec J (1998) Expression of the ErbB-neuregulin signaling network during human cerebellar development: implications for the biology of medulloblastoma. Cancer Res 58:3932–41.

Gilbertson RJ, Perry RH, Kelly PJ, Pearson AD, Lunec J (1997) Prognostic significance of HER2 and HER4 coexpression in childhood medulloblastoma. Cancer Res 57:3272–80.

Gilmour DT, Maischein HM, Nusslein-Volhard C (2002) Migration and function of a glial subtype in the vertebrate peripheral nervous system. Neuron 34:577–88.

Goodearl AD, Davis JB, Mistry K, Minghetti L, Otsu M, Waterfield MD, Stroobant P (1993) Purification of multiple forms of glial growth factor. J Biol Chem 268:18095–102.

Grimm S, Leder P (1997) An apoptosis-inducing isoform of neu differentiation factor (NDF) identified using a novel screen for dominant, apoptosis-inducing genes. J Exp Med 185:1137–42.

Grimm S, Weinstein EJ, Krane IM, Leder P (1998) Neu differentiation factor (NDF), a dominant oncogene, causes apoptosis in vitro and in vivo. J Exp Med 188:1535–9.

Grinspan JB, Marchionni MA, Reeves M, Coulaloglou M, Scherer SS (1996) Axonal interactions regulate Schwann cell apoptosis in developing peripheral nerve: neuregulin receptors and the role of neuregulins. J Neurosci 16:6107–18.

Gschwind A, Zwick E, Prenzel N, Leserer M, Ullrich A (2001) Cell communication networks: epidermal growth factor receptor transactivation as the paradigm for interreceptor signal transmission. Oncogene 20:1594–600.

Guy CT, Webster MA, Schaller M, Parsons TJ, Cardiff RD, Muller WJ (1992) Expression of the neu protooncogene in the mammary epithelium of transgenic mice induces metastatic disease. Proc Natl Acad Sci U S A 89:10578–82.

Guy PM, Platko JV, Cantley LC, Cerione RA, Carraway KL, 3rd (1994) Insect cell-expressed p180erbB3 possesses an impaired tyrosine kinase activity. Proc Natl Acad Sci U S A 91:8132–6.

Hakak Y, Walker JR, Li C, Wong WH, Davis KL, Buxbaum JD, Haroutunian V, Fienberg AA (2001) Genome-wide expression analysis reveals dysregulation of myelination-related genes in chronic schizophrenia. Proc Natl Acad Sci U S A 98:4746–51.

Halata Z, Grim M, Bauman KI (2003) Friedrich Sigmund Merkel and his "Merkel cell", morphology, development, and physiology: review and new results. Anat Rec 271A:225–39.

Hall D, Gogos JA, Karayiorgou M (2004) The contribution of three strong candidate schizophrenia susceptibility genes in demographically distinct populations. Genes Brain Behav 3:240–8.

Harari D, Tzahar E, Romano J, Shelly M, Pierce JH, Andrews GC, Yarden Y (1999) Neuregulin-4: a novel growth factor that acts through the ErbB-4 receptor tyrosine kinase. Oncogene 18:2681–9.

Hashimoto R, Straub RE, Weickert CS, Hyde TM, Kleinman JE, Weinberger DR (2004) Expression analysis of neuregulin-1 in the dorsolateral prefrontal cortex in schizophrenia. Mol Psychiatry 9:299–307.

Hebert JM, McConnell SK (2000) Targeting of cre to the Foxg1 (BF-1) locus mediates loxP recombination in the telencephalon and other developing head structures. Dev Biol 222:296–306.

Herbarth B, Pingault V, Bondurand N, Kuhlbrodt K, Hermans-Borgmeyer I, Puliti A, Lemort N, Goossens M, Wegner M (1998) Mutation of the Sry-related Sox10 gene in Dominant megacolon, a mouse model for human Hirschsprung disease. Proc Natl Acad Sci U S A 95:5161–5.

Higashiyama S, Horikawa M, Yamada K, Ichino N, Nakano N, Nakagawa T, Miyagawa J, Matsushita N, Nagatsu T, Taniguchi N, Ishiguro H (1997) A novel brain-derived member of the epidermal growth factor family that interacts with ErbB3 and ErbB4. J Biochem (Tokyo) 122:675–80.

Hippenmeyer S, Shneider NA, Birchmeier C, Burden SJ, Jessell TM, Arber S (2002) A role for neuregulin1 signaling in muscle spindle differentiation. Neuron 36:1035–49.

Holbro T, Civenni G, Hynes NE (2003) The ErbB receptors and their role in cancer progression. Exp Cell Res 284:99–110.

Holbro T, Hynes NE (2004) ErbB receptors: directing key signaling networks throughout life. Annu Rev Pharmacol Toxicol 44:195–217.

Holmes WE, Sliwkowski MX, Akita RW, Henzel WJ, Lee J, Park JW, Yansura D, Abadi N, Raab H, Lewis GD, et al. (1992) Identification of heregulin, a specific activator of p185erbB2. Science 256:1205–10.

Hong CJ, Huo SJ, Liao DL, Lee K, Wu JY, Tsai SJ (2004) Case-control and family-based association studies between the neuregulin 1 (Arg38Gln) polymorphism and schizophrenia. Neurosci Lett 366:158–61.

Hong CS, Saint-Jeannet JP (2005) Sox proteins and neural crest development. Semin Cell Dev Biol 16:694–703.

Howard B, Panchal H, McCarthy A, Ashworth A (2005) Identification of the scaramanga gene implicates Neuregulin3 in mammary gland specification. Genes Dev 19:2078–90.

Howard BA, Gusterson BA (2000a) The characterization of a mouse mutant that displays abnormal mammary gland development. Mamm Genome 11:234–7.

Howard BA, Gusterson BA (2000b) Mammary gland patterning in the AXB/BXA recombinant inbred strains of mouse. Mech Dev 91:305–9.

Howard MJ, Stanke M, Schneider C, Wu X, Rohrer H (2000) The transcription factor dHAND
    is a downstream effector of BMPs in sympathetic neuron specification. Development
    127:4073–81.

Hudziak RM, Lewis GD, Winget M, Fendly BM, Shepard HM, Ullrich A (1989) p185HER2
    monoclonal antibody has antiproliferative effects in vitro and sensitizes human breast
    tumor cells to tumor necrosis factor. Mol Cell Biol 9:1165–72.

Huotari MA, Miettinen PJ, Palgi J, Koivisto T, Ustinov J, Harari D, Yarden Y, Otonkoski T
    (2002) ErbB signaling regulates lineage determination of developing pancreatic islet cells
    in embryonic organ culture. Endocrinology 143:4437–46.

Hynes NE, Lane HA (2005) ERBB receptors and cancer: the complexity of targeted inhibitors.
    Nat Rev Cancer 5:341–54.

Hynes NE, Stern DF (1994) The biology of erbB-2/neu/HER-2 and its role in cancer. Biochim
    Biophys Acta 1198:165–84.

Ikeya M, Lee SM, Johnson JE, McMahon AP, Takada S (1997) Wnt signalling required for
    expansion of neural crest and CNS progenitors. Nature 389:966–70.

Ingham PW, McMahon AP (2001) Hedgehog signaling in animal development: paradigms
    and principles. Genes Dev 15:3059–87.

Inoue K, Tanabe Y, Lupski JR (1999) Myelin deficiencies in both the central and the peripheral
    nervous systems associated with a SOX10 mutation. Ann Neurol 46:313–8.

Iwata N, Suzuki T, Ikeda M, Kitajima T, Yamanouchi Y, Inada T, Ozaki N (2004) No association
    with the neuregulin 1 haplotype to Japanese schizophrenia. Mol Psychiatry 9:126–7.

Jannot CB, Beerli RR, Mason S, Gullick WJ, Hynes NE (1996) Intracellular expression of
    a single-chain antibody directed to the EGFR leads to growth inhibition of tumor cells.
    Oncogene 13:275–82.

Jessell TM (2000) Neuronal specification in the spinal cord: inductive signals and transcrip-
    tional codes. Nat Rev Genet 1:20–9.

Jessell TM, Siegel RE, Fischbach GD (1979) Induction of acetylcholine receptors on cultured
    skeletal muscle by a factor extracted from brain and spinal cord. Proc Natl Acad Sci U S
    A 76:5397–401.

Jessen KR, Mirsky R (2002) Signals that determine Schwann cell identity. J Anat 200:367–76.

Jessen KR, Mirsky R (2005) The origin and development of glial cells in peripheral nerves.
    Nat Rev Neurosci 6:671–82.

Jo SA, Zhu X, Marchionni MA, Burden SJ (1995) Neuregulins are concentrated at nerve-
    muscle synapses and activate ACh-receptor gene expression. Nature 373:158–61.

Jones FE, Jerry DJ, Guarino BC, Andrews GC, Stern DF (1996) Heregulin induces in vivo
    proliferation and differentiation of mammary epithelium into secretory lobuloalveoli.
    Cell Growth Differ 7:1031–8.

Jones JT, Akita RW, Sliwkowski MX (1999) Binding specificities and affinities of egf domains
    for ErbB receptors. FEBS Lett 447:227–31.

Kamachi Y, Uchikawa M, Kondoh H (2000) Pairing SOX off: with partners in the regulation
    of embryonic development. Trends Genet 16:182–7.

Kapur RP (1999) Early death of neural crest cells is responsible for total enteric aganglionosis
    in Sox10(Dom)/Sox10(Dom) mouse embryos. Pediatr Dev Pathol 2:559–69.

Kim J, Lo L, Dormand E, Anderson DJ (2003a) SOX10 maintains multipotency and inhibits
    neuronal differentiation of neural crest stem cells. Neuron 38:17–31.

Kim JY, Sun Q, Oglesbee M, Yoon SO (2003b) The role of ErbB2 signaling in the onset of
    terminal differentiation of oligodendrocytes in vivo. J Neurosci 23:5561–71.

King CR, Kraus MH, Aaronson SA (1985) Amplification of a novel v-erbB-related gene in
    a human mammary carcinoma. Science 229:974–6.

Klein R, Silos-Santiago I, Smeyne RJ, Lira SA, Brambilla R, Bryant S, Zhang L, Snider WD, Barbacid M (1994) Disruption of the neurotrophin-3 receptor gene trkC eliminates Ia muscle afferents and results in abnormal movements. Nature 368:249–51.

Knecht AK, Bronner-Fraser M (2002) Induction of the neural crest: a multigene process. Nat Rev Genet 3:453–61.

Kokai Y, Myers JN, Wada T, Brown VI, LeVea CM, Davis JG, Dobashi K, Greene MI (1989) Synergistic interaction of p185c-neu and the EGF receptor leads to transformation of rodent fibroblasts. Cell 58:287–92.

Kolodkin AL (1998) Semaphorin-mediated neuronal growth cone guidance. Prog Brain Res 117:115–32.

Kornack DR, Rakic P (2001) The generation, migration, and differentiation of olfactory neurons in the adult primate brain. Proc Natl Acad Sci U S A 98:4752–7.

Kos R, Reedy MV, Johnson RL, Erickson CA (2001) The winged-helix transcription factor FoxD3 is important for establishing the neural crest lineage and repressing melanogenesis in avian embryos. Development 128:1467–79.

Kramer R, Bucay N, Kane DJ, Martin LE, Tarpley JE, Theill LE (1996) Neuregulins with an Ig-like domain are essential for mouse myocardial and neuronal development. Proc Natl Acad Sci U S A 93:4833–8.

Krull CE, Lansford R, Gale NW, Collazo A, Marcelle C, Yancopoulos GD, Fraser SE, Bronner-Fraser M (1997) Interactions of Eph-related receptors and ligands confer rostrocaudal pattern to trunk neural crest migration. Curr Biol 7:571–80.

Kucera J, Fan G, Walro J, Copray S, Tessarollo L, Jaenisch R (1998) Neurotrophin-3 and trkC in muscle are non-essential for the development of mouse muscle spindles. Neuroreport 9:905–9.

Kuhlbrodt K, Herbarth B, Sock E, Hermans-Borgmeyer I, Wegner M (1998a) Sox10, a novel transcriptional modulator in glial cells. J Neurosci 18:237–50.

Kuhlbrodt K, Schmidt C, Sock E, Pingault V, Bondurand N, Goossens M, Wegner M (1998b) Functional analysis of Sox10 mutations found in human Waardenburg-Hirschsprung patients. J Biol Chem 273:23033–8.

Kurtz A, Zimmer A, Schnutgen F, Bruning G, Spener F, Muller T (1994) The expression pattern of a novel gene encoding brain-fatty acid binding protein correlates with neuronal and glial cell development. Development 120:2637–49.

LaBonne C, Bronner-Fraser M (2000) Snail-related transcriptional repressors are required in Xenopus for both the induction of the neural crest and its subsequent migration. Dev Biol 221:195–205.

Lai C (2005) Peripheral glia: Schwann cells in motion. Curr Biol 15:R332–4.

Lai KM, Pawson T (2000) The ShcA phosphotyrosine docking protein sensitizes cardiovascular signaling in the mouse embryo. Genes Dev 14:1132–45.

Lane PW, Liu HM (1984) Association of megacolon with a new dominant spotting gene (Dom) in the mouse. J Hered 75:435–9.

Lang D, Chen F, Milewski R, Li J, Lu MM, Epstein JA (2000) Pax3 is required for enteric ganglia formation and functions with Sox10 to modulate expression of c-ret. J Clin Invest 106:963–71.

Lang D, Epstein JA (2003) Sox10 and Pax3 physically interact to mediate activation of a conserved c-RET enhancer. Hum Mol Genet 12:937–45.

Le Douarin N, Kalcheim C (1999) The Neural Crest. Cambridge University Press.

Lee KF, Simon H, Chen H, Bates B, Hung MC, Hauser C (1995) Requirement for neuregulin receptor erbB2 in neural and cardiac development. Nature 378:394–8.

Lee KJ, Jessell TM (1999) The specification of dorsal cell fates in the vertebrate central nervous system. Annu Rev Neurosci 22:261–94.

Lefebvre V, Smits P (2005) Transcriptional control of chondrocyte fate and differentiation. Birth Defects Res C Embryo Today 75:200–12.

Leimeroth R, Lobsiger C, Lussi A, Taylor V, Suter U, Sommer L (2002) Membrane-bound neuregulin1 type III actively promotes Schwann cell differentiation of multipotent Progenitor cells. Dev Biol 246:245–58.

Lemke G (1996) Neuregulins in development. Mol Cell Neurosci 7:247–62.

Lemke GE, Brockes JP (1984) Identification and purification of glial growth factor. J Neurosci 4:75–83.

Lewandoski M (2001) Conditional control of gene expression in the mouse. Nat Rev Genet 2:743–55.

Lewis GD, Figari I, Fendly B, Wong WL, Carter P, Gorman C, Shepard HM (1993) Differential responses of human tumor cell lines to anti-p185HER2 monoclonal antibodies. Cancer Immunol Immunother 37:255–63.

Lewis GD, Lofgren JA, McMurtrey AE, Nuijens A, Fendly BM, Bauer KD, Sliwkowski MX (1996) Growth regulation of human breast and ovarian tumor cells by heregulin: Evidence for the requirement of ErbB2 as a critical component in mediating heregulin responsiveness. Cancer Res 56:1457–65.

Li L, Cleary S, Mandarano MA, Long W, Birchmeier C, Jones FE (2002) The breast proto-oncogene, HRGalpha regulates epithelial proliferation and lobuloalveolar development in the mouse mammary gland. Oncogene 21:4900–7.

Li T, Stefansson H, Gudfinnsson E, Cai G, Liu X, Murray RM, Steinthorsdottir V, Januel D, Gudnadottir VG, Petursson H, Ingason A, Gulcher JR, Stefansson K, Collier DA (2004) Identification of a novel neuregulin 1 at-risk haplotype in Han schizophrenia Chinese patients, but no association with the Icelandic/Scottish risk haplotype. Mol Psychiatry 9:698–704.

Liem KF, Jr., Tremml G, Jessell TM (1997) A role for the roof plate and its resident TGFbeta-related proteins in neuronal patterning in the dorsal spinal cord. Cell 91:127–38.

Liem KF, Jr., Tremml G, Roelink H, Jessell TM (1995) Dorsal differentiation of neural plate cells induced by BMP-mediated signals from epidermal ectoderm. Cell 82:969–79.

Lin W, Sanchez HB, Deerinck T, Morris JK, Ellisman M, Lee KF (2000) Aberrant development of motor axons and neuromuscular synapses in erbB2-deficient mice. Proc Natl Acad Sci U S A 97:1299–304.

Liu X, Hwang H, Cao L, Buckland M, Cunningham A, Chen J, Chien KR, Graham RM, Zhou M (1998) Domain-specific gene disruption reveals critical regulation of neuregulin signaling by its cytoplasmic tail. Proc Natl Acad Sci U S A 95:13024–9.

Liu Y, Ford B, Mann MA, Fischbach GD (2001) Neuregulins increase alpha7 nicotinic acetylcholine receptors and enhance excitatory synaptic transmission in GABAergic interneurons of the hippocampus. J Neurosci 21:5660–9.

Lobsiger CS, Taylor V, Suter U (2002) The early life of a Schwann cell. Biol Chem 383:245–53.

Lohmueller KE, Pearce CL, Pike M, Lander ES, Hirschhorn JN (2003) Meta-analysis of genetic association studies supports a contribution of common variants to susceptibility to common disease. Nat Genet 33:177–82.

Long W, Wagner KU, Lloyd KC, Binart N, Shillingford JM, Hennighausen L, Jones FE (2003) Impaired differentiation and lactational failure of Erbb4-deficient mammary glands identify ERBB4 as an obligate mediator of STAT5. Development 130:5257–68.

Longart M, Liu Y, Karavanova I, Buonanno A (2004) Neuregulin-2 is developmentally regulated and targeted to dendrites of central neurons. J Comp Neurol 472:156–72.

Luetteke NC, Qiu TH, Fenton SE, Troyer KL, Riedel RF, Chang A, Lee DC (1999) Targeted inactivation of the EGF and amphiregulin genes reveals distinct roles for EGF receptor ligands in mouse mammary gland development. Development 126:2739–50.

Luskin MB (1993) Restricted proliferation and migration of postnatally generated neurons derived from the forebrain subventricular zone. Neuron 11:173–89.

Lyons DA, Pogoda HM, Voas MG, Woods IG, Diamond B, Nix R, Arana N, Jacobs J, Talbot WS (2005) erbb3 and erbb2 are essential for Schwann cell migration and myelination in zebrafish. Curr Biol 15:513–24.

Ma Q, Fode C, Guillemot F, Anderson DJ (1999) Neurogenin1 and neurogenin2 control two distinct waves of neurogenesis in developing dorsal root ganglia. Genes Dev 13:1717–28.

Mahanthappa NK, Anton ES, Matthew WD (1996) Glial growth factor 2, a soluble neuregulin, directly increases Schwann cell motility and indirectly promotes neurite outgrowth. J Neurosci 16:4673–83.

Maier M, Berger P, Suter U (2002) Understanding Schwann cell-neurone interactions: the key to Charcot-Marie-Tooth disease? J Anat 200:357–66.

Marchant L, Linker C, Ruiz P, Guerrero N, Mayor R (1998) The inductive properties of mesoderm suggest that the neural crest cells are specified by a BMP gradient. Dev Biol 198:319–29.

Marchionni MA, Goodearl AD, Chen MS, Bermingham MO, Kirk C, Hendricks M, Danehy F, Misumi D, Sudhalter J, Kobayashi K, et al 1993. Glial growth factors are alternatively spliced erbB2 ligands expressed in the nervous system. Nature 362:312–8.

Marone R, Hess D, Dankort D, Muller WJ, Hynes NE, Badache A (2004) Memo mediates ErbB2-driven cell motility. Nat Cell Biol 6:515–22.

Martin P, Lewis J (1989) Origins of the neurovascular bundle: interactions between developing nerves and blood vessels in embryonic chick skin. Int J Dev Biol 33:379–87.

Massague J, Blain SW, Lo RS (2000) TGFbeta signaling in growth control, cancer, and heritable disorders. Cell 103:295–309.

Matsuo S, Ichikawa H, Silos-Santiago I, Arends JJ, Henderson TA, Kiyomiya K, Kurebe M, Jacquin MF (2000) Proprioceptive afferents survive in the masseter muscle of trkC knockout mice. Neuroscience 95:209–16.

Meier C, Parmantier E, Brennan A, Mirsky R, Jessen KR (1999) Developing Schwann cells acquire the ability to survive without axons by establishing an autocrine circuit involving insulin-like growth factor, neurotrophin-3, and platelet-derived growth factor-BB. J Neurosci 19:3847–59.

Meintanis S, Thomaidou D, Jessen KR, Mirsky R, Matsas R (2001) The neuron-glia signal beta-neuregulin promotes Schwann cell motility via the MAPK pathway. Glia 34:39–51.

Meulemans D, Bronner-Fraser M (2004) Gene-regulatory interactions in neural crest evolution and development. Dev Cell 7:291–9.

Meyer D, Birchmeier C (1994) Distinct isoforms of neuregulin are expressed in mesenchymal and neuronal cells during mouse development. Proc Natl Acad Sci U S A 91:1064–8.

Meyer D, Birchmeier C (1995) Multiple essential functions of neuregulin in development. Nature 378:386–90.

Meyer D, Yamaai T, Garratt A, Riethmacher-Sonneberg E, Kane D, Theill L, Birchmeier C (1997) Isoform specific expression and function of neuregulin. Development 124:3575–3586.

Michailov GV, Sereda MW, Brinkmann BG, Fischer TM, Haug B, Birchmeier C, Role L, Lai C, Schwab MH, Nave KA (2004) Axonal neuregulin-1 regulates myelin sheath thickness. Science 304:700–3.

Mollaaghababa R, Pavan WJ (2003) The importance of having your SOX on: role of SOX10 in the development of neural crest-derived melanocytes and glia. Oncogene 22:3024–34.

Morris JK, Lin W, Hauser C, Marchuk Y, Getman D, Lee KF (1999) Rescue of the cardiac defect in ErbB2 mutant mice reveals essential roles of ErbB2 in peripheral nervous system development. Neuron 23:273–83.

Morrison SJ, Perez SE, Qiao Z, Verdi JM, Hicks C, Weinmaster G, Anderson DJ (2000) Transient Notch activation initiates an irreversible switch from neurogenesis to gliogenesis by neural crest stem cells. Cell 101:499–510.

Moscoso LM, Chu GC, Gautam M, Noakes PG, Merlie JP, Sanes JR (1995) Synapse-associated expression of an acetylcholine receptor-inducing protein, ARIA/heregulin, and its putative receptors, ErbB2 and ErbB3, in developing mammalian muscle. Dev Biol 172:158–69.

Moury JD, Jacobson AG (1990) The origins of neural crest cells in the axolotl. Dev Biol 141:243–53.

Mukouyama YS, Shin D, Britsch S, Taniguchi M, Anderson DJ (2002) Sensory nerves determine the pattern of arterial differentiation and blood vessel branching in the skin. Cell 109:693–705.

Muller U (1999) Ten years of gene targeting: targeted mouse mutants, from vector design to phenotype analysis. Mech Dev 82:3–21.

Muller WJ, Sinn E, Pattengale PK, Wallace R, Leder P (1988) Single-step induction of mammary adenocarcinoma in transgenic mice bearing the activated c-neu oncogene. Cell 54:105–15.

Muss HB, Thor AD, Berry DA, Kute T, Liu ET, Koerner F, Cirrincione CT, Budman DR, Wood WC, Barcos M et al. (1994) c-erbB-2 expression and response to adjuvant therapy in women with node-positive early breast cancer. N Engl J Med 330:1260–6.

Nebigil CG, Choi DS, Dierich A, Hickel P, Le Meur M, Messaddeq N, Launay JM, Maroteaux L (2000) Serotonin 2B receptor is required for heart development. Proc Natl Acad Sci U S A 97:9508–13.

Negro A, Brar BK, Lee KF (2004) Essential roles of Her2/erbB2 in cardiac development and function. Recent Prog Horm Res 59:1–12.

Nieto MA, Sargent MG, Wilkinson DG, Cooke J (1994) Control of cell behavior during vertebrate development by Slug, a zinc finger gene. Science 264:835–9.

Nikitin A, Ballering LA, Lyons J, Rajewsky MF (1991) Early mutation of the neu (erbB-2) gene during ethylnitrosourea-induced oncogenesis in the rat Schwann cell lineage. Proc Natl Acad Sci U S A 88:9939–43.

Ogiso H, Ishitani R, Nureki O, Fukai S, Yamanaka M, Kim JH, Saito K, Sakamoto A, Inoue M, Shirouzu M, Yokoyama S (2002) Crystal structure of the complex of human epidermal growth factor and receptor extracellular domains. Cell 110:775–87.

Okada M, Corfas G (2004) Neuregulin1 downregulates postsynaptic GABAA receptors at the hippocampal inhibitory synapse. Hippocampus 14:337–44.

Olayioye MA, Neve RM, Lane HA, Hynes NE (2000) The ErbB signaling network: receptor heterodimerization in development and cancer. Embo J 19:3159–67.

Owen MJ, Craddock N, O'Donovan MC (2005) Schizophrenia: genes at last? Trends Genet 21:518–25.

Ozaki M (2001) Neuregulins and the shaping of synapses. Neuroscientist 7:146–54.

Ozaki M, Sasner M, Yano R, Lu HS, Buonanno A (1997) Neuregulin-beta induces expression of an NMDA-receptor subunit. Nature 390:691–4.

Ozcelik C, Erdmann B, Pilz B, Wettschureck N, Britsch S, Hubner N, Chien KR, Birchmeier C, Garratt AN (2002) Conditional mutation of the ErbB2 (HER2) receptor in cardiomyocytes leads to dilated cardiomyopathy. Proc Natl Acad Sci U S A 99:8880–5.

Papadatos GA, Wallerstein PM, Head CE, Ratcliff R, Brady PA, Benndorf K, Saumarez RC, Trezise AE, Huang CL, Vandenberg JI, Colledge WH, Grace AA (2002) Slowed conduction and ventricular tachycardia after targeted disruption of the cardiac sodium channel gene Scn5a. Proc Natl Acad Sci U S A 99:6210–5.

Paratore C, Goerich DE, Suter U, Wegner M, Sommer L (2001) Survival and glial fate acquisition of neural crest cells are regulated by an interplay between the transcription factor Sox10 and extrinsic combinatorial signaling. Development 128:3949–61.

Pegram MD, Lipton A, Hayes DF, Weber BL, Baselga JM, Tripathy D, Baly D, Baughman SA, Twaddell T, Glaspy JA, Slamon DJ (1998) Phase II study of receptor-enhanced chemosensitivity using recombinant humanized anti-p185HER2/neu monoclonal antibody plus cisplatin in patients with HER2/neu-overexpressing metastatic breast cancer refractory to chemotherapy treatment. J Clin Oncol 16:2659–71.

Peifer M, Polakis P (2000) Wnt signaling in oncogenesis and embryogenesis–a look outside the nucleus. Science 287:1606–9.

Peirano RI, Goerich DE, Riethmacher D, Wegner M (2000) Protein zero gene expression is regulated by the glial transcription factor Sox10. Mol Cell Biol 20:3198–209.

Peirano RI, Wegner M (2000) The glial transcription factor Sox10 binds to DNA both as monomer and dimer with different functional consequences. Nucleic Acids Res 28:3047–55.

Peles E, Ben LR, Tzahar E, Liu N, Wen D, Yarden Y (1993) Cell-type specific interaction of Neu differentiation factor (NDF/heregulin) with Neu/HER-2 suggests complex ligand-receptor relationships. Embo J. 12:961–71.

Pevny LH, Lovell-Badge R (1997) Sox genes find their feet. Curr Opin Genet Dev 7:338–44.

Pingault V, Bondurand N, Kuhlbrodt K, Goerich DE, Prehu MO, Puliti A, Herbarth B, Hermans-Borgmeyer I, Legius E, Matthijs G, Amiel J, Lyonnet S, Ceccherini I, Romeo G, Smith JC, Read AP, Wegner M, Goossens M (1998) SOX10 mutations in patients with Waardenburg-Hirschsprung disease. Nat Genet 18:171–3.

Pingault V, Bondurand N, Le Caignec C, Tardieu S, Lemort N, Dubourg O, Le Guern E, Goossens M, Boespflug-Tanguy O (2001) The SOX10 transcription factor: evaluation as a candidate gene for central and peripheral hereditary myelin disorders. J Neurol 248:496–9.

Pingault V, Guiochon-Mantel A, Bondurand N, Faure C, Lacroix C, Lyonnet S, Goossens M, Landrieu P (2000) Peripheral neuropathy with hypomyelination, chronic intestinal pseudo-obstruction and deafness: a developmental "neural crest syndrome" related to a SOX10 mutation. Ann Neurol 48:671–6.

Plowman GD, Green JM, Culouscou JM, Carlton GW, Rothwell VM, Buckley S (1993) Heregulin induces tyrosine phosphorylation of HER4/p180erbB4. Nature 366:473–5.

Poliakov A, Cotrina M, Wilkinson DG (2004) Diverse roles of eph receptors and ephrins in the regulation of cell migration and tissue assembly. Dev Cell 7:465–80.

Ponomareva ON, Ma H, Dakour R, Raabe TD, Lai C, Rimer M (2005) Stimulation of acetylcholine receptor transcription by neuregulin-2 requires an N-box response element and is regulated by alternative splicing. Neuroscience 134:495–503.

Prenzel N, Fischer OM, Streit S, Hart S, Ullrich A (2001) The epidermal growth factor receptor family as a central element for cellular signal transduction and diversification. Endocr Relat Cancer 8:11–31.

Prenzel N, Zwick E, Daub H, Leserer M, Abraham R, Wallasch C, Ullrich A (1999) EGF receptor transactivation by G-protein-coupled receptors requires metalloproteinase cleavage of proHB-EGF. Nature 402:884–8.

Press MF, Bernstein L, Thomas PA, Meisner LF, Zhou JY, Ma Y, Hung G, Robinson RA, Harris C, El-Naggar A, Slamon DJ, Phillips RN, Ross JS, Wolman SR, Flom KJ (1997) HER-2/neu gene amplification characterized by fluorescence in situ hybridization: poor prognosis in node-negative breast carcinomas. J Clin Oncol 15:2894–904.

Price SR, De Marco Garcia NV, Ranscht B, Jessell TM (2002) Regulation of motor neuron pool sorting by differential expression of type II cadherins. Cell 109:205–16.

Pusch C, Hustert E, Pfeifer D, Sudbeck P, Kist R, Roe B, Wang Z, Balling R, Blin N, Scherer G (1998) The SOX10/Sox10 gene from human and mouse: sequence, expression, and transactivation by the encoded HMG domain transcription factor. Hum Genet 103:115–23.

Raff MC, Abney E, Brockes JP, Hornby-Smith A (1978) Schwann cell growth factors. Cell 15:813–22.

Ramsauer VP, Carraway CA, Salas PJ, Carraway KL (2003) Muc4/sialomucin complex, the intramembrane ErbB2 ligand, translocates ErbB2 to the apical surface in polarized epithelial cells. J Biol Chem 278:30142–7.

Reissmann E, Ernsberger U, Francis-West PH, Rueger D, Brickell PM, Rohrer H (1996) Involvement of bone morphogenetic protein-4 and bone morphogenetic protein-7 in the differentiation of the adrenergic phenotype in developing sympathetic neurons. Development 122:2079–88.

Rieff HI, Raetzman LT, Sapp DW, Yeh HH, Siegel RE, Corfas G (1999) Neuregulin induces GABA(A) receptor subunit expression and neurite outgrowth in cerebellar granule cells. J Neurosci 19:10757–66.

Riethmacher D, Sonnenberg RE, Brinkmann V, Yamaai T, Lewin GR, Birchmeier C (1997) Severe neuropathies in mice with targeted mutations in the ErbB3 receptor. Nature 389:725–30.

Rimer M, Cohen I, Lomo T, Burden SJ, McMahan UJ (1998) Neuregulins and erbB receptors at neuromuscular junctions and at agrin-induced postsynaptic-like apparatus in skeletal muscle. Mol Cell Neurosci 12:1–15.

Rimer M, Prieto AL, Weber JL, Colasante C, Ponomareva O, Fromm L, Schwab MH, Lai C, Burden SJ (2004) Neuregulin-2 is synthesized by motor neurons and terminal Schwann cells and activates acetylcholine receptor transcription in muscle cells expressing ErbB4. Mol Cell Neurosci 26:271–81.

Rio C, Rieff HI, Qi P, Khurana TS, Corfas G (1997) Neuregulin and erbB receptors play a critical role in neuronal migration. Neuron 19:39–50.

Ross JS, Fletcher JA (1998) The HER-2/neu oncogene in breast cancer: prognostic factor, predictive factor, and target for therapy. Stem Cells 16:413–28.

Salzer JL, Bunge RP, Glaser L (1980) Studies of Schwann cell proliferation. III. Evidence for the surface localization of the neurite mitogen. J Cell Biol 84:767–78.

Sandrock AW, Jr., Dryer SE, Rosen KM, Gozani SN, Kramer R, Theill LE, Fischbach GD (1997) Maintenance of acetylcholine receptor number by neuregulins at the neuromuscular junction in vivo. Science 276:599–603.

Sanes JR, Lichtman JW (1999) Development of the vertebrate neuromuscular junction. Ann. Rev. Neurosci. 22:389–442.

Sanes JR, Lichtman JW (2001) Induction, assembly, maturation and maintenance of a postsynaptic apparatus. Nat Rev Neurosci 2:791–805.

Scarisbrick IA, Jones EG, Isackson PJ (1993) Coexpression of mRNAs for NGF, BDNF, and NT-3 in the cardiovascular system of the pre- and postnatal rat. J Neurosci 13:875–93.

Schlessinger J (2000) Cell signaling by receptor tyrosine kinases. Cell 103:211–25.

Schmid RS, McGrath B, Berechid BE, Boyles B, Marchionni M, Sestan N, Anton ES (2003) Neuregulin 1-erbB2 signaling is required for the establishment of radial glia and their transformation into astrocytes in cerebral cortex. Proc Natl Acad Sci U S A 100:4251–6.

Schmucker J, Ader M, Brockschnieder D, Brodarac A, Bartsch U, Riethmacher D (2003) erbB3 is dispensable for oligodendrocyte development in vitro and in vivo. Glia 44:67–75.

Schneider C, Wicht H, Enderich J, Wegner M, Rohrer H (1999) Bone morphogenetic proteins are required in vivo for the generation of sympathetic neurons. Neuron 24:861–70.

Schuchardt A, D'Agati V, Larsson-Blomberg L, Costantini F, Pachnis V (1994) Defects in the kidney and enteric nervous system of mice lacking the tyrosine kinase receptor Ret. Nature 367:380–3.

Schuchardt A, D'Agati V, Larsson-Blomberg L, Costantini F, Pachnis V (1995) RET-deficient mice: an animal model for Hirschsprung's disease and renal agenesis. J Intern Med 238:327–32.

Seals DF, Courtneidge SA (2003) The ADAMs family of metalloproteases: multidomain proteins with multiple functions. Genes Dev 17:7–30.

Seidman A, Hudis C, Pierri MK, Shak S, Paton V, Ashby M, Murphy M, Stewart SJ, Keefe D (2002) Cardiac dysfunction in the trastuzumab clinical trials experience. J Clin Oncol 20:1215–21.

Selleck MA, Bronner-Fraser M (1995) Origins of the avian neural crest: the role of neural plate-epidermal interactions. Development 121:525–38.

Shah NM, Groves AK, Anderson DJ (1996) Alternative neural crest cell fates are instructively promoted by TGFbeta superfamily members. Cell 85:331–43.

Sheng Z, Wu K, Carraway KL, Fregien N (1992) Molecular cloning of the transmembrane component of the 13762 mammary adenocarcinoma sialomucin complex. A new member of the epidermal growth factor superfamily. J Biol Chem 267:16341–6.

Shima DT, Mailhos C (2000) Vascular developmental biology: getting nervous. Curr Opin Genet Dev 10:536–42.

Slamon DJ, Clark GM, Wong SG, Levin WJ, Ullrich A, McGuire WL (1987) Human breast cancer: correlation of relapse and survival with amplification of the HER-2/neu oncogene. Science 235:177–82.

Slamon DJ, Godolphin W, Jones LA, Holt JA, Wong SG, Keith DE, Levin WJ, Stuart SG, Udove J, Ullrich A et al. (1989) Studies of the HER-2/neu proto-oncogene in human breast and ovarian cancer. Science 244:707–12.

Slamon DJ, Leyland-Jones B, Shak S, Fuchs H, Paton V, Bajamonde A, Fleming T, Eiermann W, Wolter J, Pegram M, Baselga J, Norton L (2001) Use of chemotherapy plus a monoclonal antibody against HER2 for metastatic breast cancer that overexpresses HER2. N Engl J Med 344:783–92.

Sliwkowski MX, Lofgren JA, Lewis GD, Hotaling TE, Fendly BM, Fox JA (1999) Nonclinical studies addressing the mechanism of action of trastuzumab (Herceptin). Semin Oncol 26:60–70.

Sliwkowski MX, Schaefer G, Akita RW, Lofgren JA, Fitzpatrick VD, Nuijens A, Fendly BM, Cerione RA, Vandlen RL, Carraway KR (1994) Coexpression of erbB2 and erbB3 proteins reconstitutes a high affinity receptor for heregulin. J Biol. Chem. 269:14661–5.

Sonnenberg-Riethmacher E, Miehe M, Stolt CC, Goerich DE, Wegner M, Riethmacher D (2001) Development and degeneration of dorsal root ganglia in the absence of the HMG-domain transcription factor Sox10. Mech Dev 109:253–65.

Southard-Smith EM, Angrist M, Ellison JS, Agarwala R, Baxevanis AD, Chakravarti A, Pavan WJ (1999) The Sox10(Dom) mouse: modeling the genetic variation of Waardenburg-Shah (WS4) syndrome. Genome Res 9:215–25.

Southard-Smith EM, Kos L, Pavan WJ (1998) Sox10 mutation disrupts neural crest development in Dom Hirschsprung mouse model. Nat Genet 18:60–4.

Spokony RF, Aoki Y, Saint-Germain N, Magner-Fink E, Saint-Jeannet JP (2002) The transcription factor Sox9 is required for cranial neural crest development in Xenopus. Development 129:421–32.

Stefansson H, Sigurdsson E, Steinthorsdottir V, Bjornsdottir S, Sigmundsson T, Ghosh S, Brynjolfsson J, Gunnarsdottir S, Ivarsson O, Chou TT, Hjaltason O, Birgisdottir B, Jonsson H, Gudnadottir VG, Gudmundsdottir E, Bjornsson A, Ingvarsson B, Ingason A, Sigfusson S, Hardardottir H, Harvey RP, Lai D, Zhou M, Brunner D, Mutel V, Gonzalo A, Lemke G, Sainz J, Johannesson G, Andresson T, Gudbjartsson D, Manolescu A, Frigge ML, Gurney ME, Kong A, Gulcher JR, Petursson H, Stefansson K (2002) Neuregulin 1 and susceptibility to schizophrenia. Am J Hum Genet 71:877–92.

Stefansson H, Steinthorsdottir V, Thorgeirsson TE, Gulcher JR, Stefansson K (2004) Neuregulin 1 and schizophrenia. Ann Med 36:62–71.

Steiner H, Blum M, Kitai ST, Fedi P (1999) Differential expression of ErbB3 and ErbB4 neuregulin receptors in dopamine neurons and forebrain areas of the adult rat. Exp Neurol 159:494–503.

Stolt CC, Lommes P, Sock E, Chaboissier MC, Schedl A, Wegner M (2003) The Sox9 transcription factor determines glial fate choice in the developing spinal cord. Genes Dev 17:1677–89.

Suter U, Scherer SS (2003) Disease mechanisms in inherited neuropathies. Nat Rev Neurosci 4:714–26.

Syroid DE, Maycox PR, Burrola PG, Liu N, Wen D, Lee KF, Lemke G, Kilpatrick TJ (1996) Cell death in the Schwann cell lineage and its regulation by neuregulin. Proc Natl Acad Sci U S A 93:9229–34.

Syroid DE, Zorick TS, Arbet-Engels C, Kilpatrick TJ, Eckhart W, Lemke G (1999) A role for insulin-like growth factor-I in the regulation of Schwann cell survival. J Neurosci 19:2059–68.

Szeder V, Grim M, Halata Z, Sieber-Blum M (2003) Neural crest origin of mammalian Merkel cells. Dev Biol 253:258–63.

Talmage DA, Role LW (2004) Multiple personalities of neuregulin gene family members. J Comp Neurol 472:134–9.

Tang JX, Chen WY, He G, Zhou J, Gu NF, Feng GY, He L (2004) Polymorphisms within 5' end of the Neuregulin 1 gene are genetically associated with schizophrenia in the Chinese population. Mol Psychiatry 9:11–2.

Taniguchi M, Yuasa S, Fujisawa H, Naruse I, Saga S, Mishina M, Yagi T (1997) Disruption of semaphorin III/D gene causes severe abnormality in peripheral nerve projection. Neuron 19:519–30.

Taveggia C, Zanazzi G, Petrylak A, Yano H, Rosenbluth J, Einheber S, Xu X, Esper RM, Loeb JA, Shrager P, Chao MV, Falls DL, Role L, Salzer JL (2005) Neuregulin-1 type III determines the ensheathment fate of axons. Neuron 47:681–94.

Thiselton DL, Webb BT, Neale BM, Ribble RC, O'Neill FA, Walsh D, Riley BP, Kendler KS (2004) No evidence for linkage or association of neuregulin-1 (NRG1) with disease in the Irish study of high-density schizophrenia families (ISHDSF). Mol Psychiatry 9:777–83; image 729.

Thomas SA, Matsumoto AM, Palmiter RD (1995) Noradrenaline is essential for mouse fetal development. Nature 374:643–6.

Tidcombe H, Jackson-Fisher A, Mathers K, Stern DF, Gassmann M, Golding JP (2003) Neural and mammary gland defects in ErbB4 knockout mice genetically rescued from embryonic lethality. Proc Natl Acad Sci U S A 100:8281–6.

Tkachev D, Mimmack ML, Ryan MM, Wayland M, Freeman T, Jones PB, Starkey M, Webster MJ, Yolken RH, Bahn S (2003) Oligodendrocyte dysfunction in schizophrenia and bipolar disorder. Lancet 362:798–805.

Touraine RL, Attie-Bitach T, Manceau E, Korsch E, Sarda P, Pingault V, Encha-Razavi F, Pelet A, Auge J, Nivelon-Chevallier A, Holschneider AM, Munnes M, Doerfler W, Goossens M, Munnich A, Vekemans M, Lyonnet S (2000) Neurological phenotype in Waardenburg syndrome type 4 correlates with novel SOX10 truncating mutations and expression in developing brain. Am J Hum Genet 66:1496–503.

Tourtellotte WG, Milbrandt J (1998) Sensory ataxia and muscle spindle agenesis in mice lacking the transcription factor Egr3. Nat Genet 20:87–91.

Trinidad JC, Fischbach GD, Cohen JB (2000) The Agrin/MuSK signaling pathway is spatially segregated from the neuregulin/ErbB receptor signaling pathway at the neuromuscular junction. J Neurosci 20:8762–70.

Tzahar E, Levkowitz G, Karunagaran D, Yi L, Peles E, Lavi S, Chang D, Liu NL, Yayon A, Wen DZ, Yarden Y (1994) Erbb-3 and erbb-4 function as the respective low and high affinity receptors of all neu differentiation factor heregulin isoforms. Journal of Biological Chemistry 269:25226–25233.

Ueda H, Oikawa A, Nakamura A, Terasawa F, Kawagishi K, Moriizumi T (2005) Neuregulin receptor ErbB2 localization at T-tubule in cardiac and skeletal muscle. J Histochem Cytochem 53:87–91.

Urban S, Lee JR, Freeman M (2002) A family of Rhomboid intramembrane proteases activates all Drosophila membrane-tethered EGF ligands. Embo J 21:4277–86.

Vartanian T, Corfas G, Li Y, Fischbach GD, Stefansson K (1994) A role for the acetylcholine receptor-inducing protein ARIA in oligodendrocyte development. Proc Natl Acad Sci U S A 91:11626–30.

Vartanian T, Fischbach G, Miller R (1999) Failure of spinal cord oligodendrocyte development in mice lacking neuregulin. Proc Natl Acad Sci U S A 96:731–5.

Volk T (1999) Singling out Drosophila tendon cells: a dialogue between two distinct cell types. Trends Genet 15:448–53.

Wakamatsu Y, Maynard TM, Weston JA (2000) Fate determination of neural crest cells by NOTCH-mediated lateral inhibition and asymmetrical cell division during gangliogenesis. Development 127:2811–21.

Wallasch C, Weiss FU, Niederfellner G, Jallal B, Issing W, Ullrich A (1995) Heregulin-dependent regulation of her2/neu oncogenic signaling by heterodimerization with her3. Embo Journal 14:4267–4275.

Wang HU, Anderson DJ (1997) Eph family transmembrane ligands can mediate repulsive guidance of trunk neural crest migration and motor axon outgrowth. Neuron 18:383–96.

Wang JY, Frenzel KE, Wen D, Falls DL (1998) Transmembrane neuregulins interact with LIM kinase 1, a cytoplasmic protein kinase implicated in development of visuospatial cognition. J Biol Chem 273:20525–34.

Wang S, Barres BA (2000) Up a notch: instructing gliogenesis. Neuron 27:197–200.

Wegner M (1999) From head to toes: the multiple facets of Sox proteins. Nucleic Acids Res 27:1409–20.

Wegner M, Stolt CC (2005) From stem cells to neurons and glia: a Soxist's view of neural development. Trends Neurosci 28:583–8.

Weiner JA, Chun J (1999) Schwann cell survival mediated by the signaling phospholipid lysophosphatidic acid. Proc Natl Acad Sci U S A 96:5233–8.

Weinmaster G, Roberts VJ, Lemke G (1991) A homolog of Drosophila Notch expressed during mammalian development. Development 113:199–205.

Weinstein EJ, Leder P (2000) The extracellular region of heregulin is sufficient to promote mammary gland proliferation and tumorigenesis but not apoptosis. Cancer Res 60:3856–61.

Wen D, Peles E, Cupples R, Suggs SV, Bacus SS, Luo Y, Trail G, Hu S, Silbiger SM, Levy RB et al. (1992) Neu differentiation factor: a transmembrane glycoprotein containing an EGF domain and an immunoglobulin homology unit. Cell 69:559-72.

Wilson M, Koopman P (2002) Matching SOX: partner proteins and co-factors of the SOX family of transcriptional regulators. Curr Opin Genet Dev 12:441-6.

Woldeyesus MT, Britsch S, Riethmacher D, Xu L, Sonnenberg-Riethmacher E, Abou-Rebyeh F, Harvey R, Caroni P, Birchmeier C (1999) Peripheral nervous system defects in erbB2 mutants following genetic rescue of heart development. Genes Dev 13:2538-48.

Wolpowitz D, Mason TB, Dietrich P, Mendelsohn M, Talmage DA, Role LW (2000) Cysteine-rich domain isoforms of the neuregulin-1 gene are required for maintenance of peripheral synapses. Neuron 25:79-91.

Yamamoto Y, Livet J, Pollock RA, Garces A, Arce V, deLapeyriere O, Henderson CE (1997) Hepatocyte growth factor (HGF/SF) is a muscle-derived survival factor for a subpopulation of embryonic motoneurons. Development 124:2903-13.

Yamauchi T, Ueki K, Tobe K, Tamemoto H, Sekine N, Wada M, Honjo M, Takahashi M, Takahashi T, Hirai H, Tushima T, Akanuma Y, Fujita T, Komuro I, Yazaki Y, Kadowaki T (1997) Tyrosine phosphorylation of the EGF receptor by the kinase Jak2 is induced by growth hormone. Nature 390:91-6.

Yamauchi T, Yamauchi N, Ueki K, Sugiyama T, Waki H, Miki H, Tobe K, Matsuda S, Tsushima T, Yamamoto T, Fujita T, Taketani Y, Fukayama M, Kimura S, Yazaki Y, Nagai R, Kadowaki T (2000) Constitutive tyrosine phosphorylation of ErbB-2 via Jak2 by autocrine secretion of prolactin in human breast cancer. J Biol Chem 275:33937-44.

Yan Y, Shirakabe K, Werb Z (2002) The metalloprotease Kuzbanian (ADAM10) mediates the transactivation of EGF receptor by G protein-coupled receptors. J Cell Biol 158:221-6.

Yang JZ, Si TM, Ruan Y, Ling YS, Han YH, Wang XL, Zhou M, Zhang HY, Kong QM, Liu C, Zhang DR, Yu YQ, Liu SZ, Ju GZ, Shu L, Ma DL, Zhang D (2003) Association study of neuregulin 1 gene with schizophrenia. Mol Psychiatry 8:706-9.

Yang X, Arber S, William C, Li L, Tanabe Y, Jessell TM, Birchmeier C, Burden SJ (2001) Patterning of muscle acetylcholine receptor gene expression in the absence of motor innervation. Neuron 30:399-410.

Yang X, Kuo Y, Devay P, Yu C, Role L (1998) A cysteine-rich isoform of neuregulin controls the level of expression of neuronal nicotinic receptor channels during synaptogenesis. Neuron 20:255-70.

Yang Y, Spitzer E, Meyer D, Sachs M, Niemann C, Hartmann G, Weidner KM, Birchmeier C, Birchmeier W (1995) Sequential requirement of hepatocyte growth factor and neuregulin in the morphogenesis and differentiation of the mammary gland. J Cell Biol 131:215-26.

Yarden, and Y Sliwkowski MX (2001) Untangling the ErbB signalling network. Nat Rev Mol Cell Biol 2:127-37.

Yarnitzky T, Min L, Volk T (1997) The Drosophila neuregulin homolog Vein mediates inductive interactions between myotubes and their epidermal attachment cells. Genes Dev 11:2691-700.

Yau HJ, Wang HF, Lai C, Liu FC (2003) Neural development of the neuregulin receptor ErbB4 in the cerebral cortex and the hippocampus: preferential expression by interneurons tangentially migrating from the ganglionic eminences. Cereb Cortex 13:252-64.

Zelena J (1994) Nerves and Mechanoreceptors: The Role of innervation in the Development and Maintenance of Mammalian Mechanoreceptors. Chapman & Hall, London.

Zhang D, Sliwkowski MX, Mark M, Frantz G, Akita R, Sun Y, Hillan K, Crowley C, Brush J, Godowski PJ (1997) Neuregulin-3 (NRG3): a novel neural tissue-enriched protein that binds and activates ErbB4. Proc Natl Acad Sci U S A 94:9562-7.

Zhao X, Shi Y, Tang J, Tang R, Yu L, Gu N, Feng G, Zhu S, Liu H, Xing Y, Zhao S, Sang H, Guan Y, St Clair D, He L (2004) A case control and family based association study of the neuregulin1 gene and schizophrenia. J Med Genet 41:31–4.

Zhao YY, Sawyer DR, Baliga RR, Opel DJ, Han X, Marchionni MA, Kelly RA (1998) Neuregulins promote survival and growth of cardiac myocytes. Persistence of ErbB2 and ErbB4 expression in neonatal and adult ventricular myocytes. J Biol Chem 273:10261–9.

Zhou QY, Quaife CJ, Palmiter RD (1995) Targeted disruption of the tyrosine hydroxylase gene reveals that catecholamines are required for mouse fetal development. Nature 374:640–3.

Zhu X, Lai C, Thomas S, Burden SJ (1995) Neuregulin receptors, erbB3 and erbB4, are localized at neuromuscular synapses. Embo J 14:5842–8.

# Subject Index

13749454R00051

Made in the USA
Lexington, KY
22 February 2012